NATURALLY BEAUTIFUL

The Complete Beauty Book

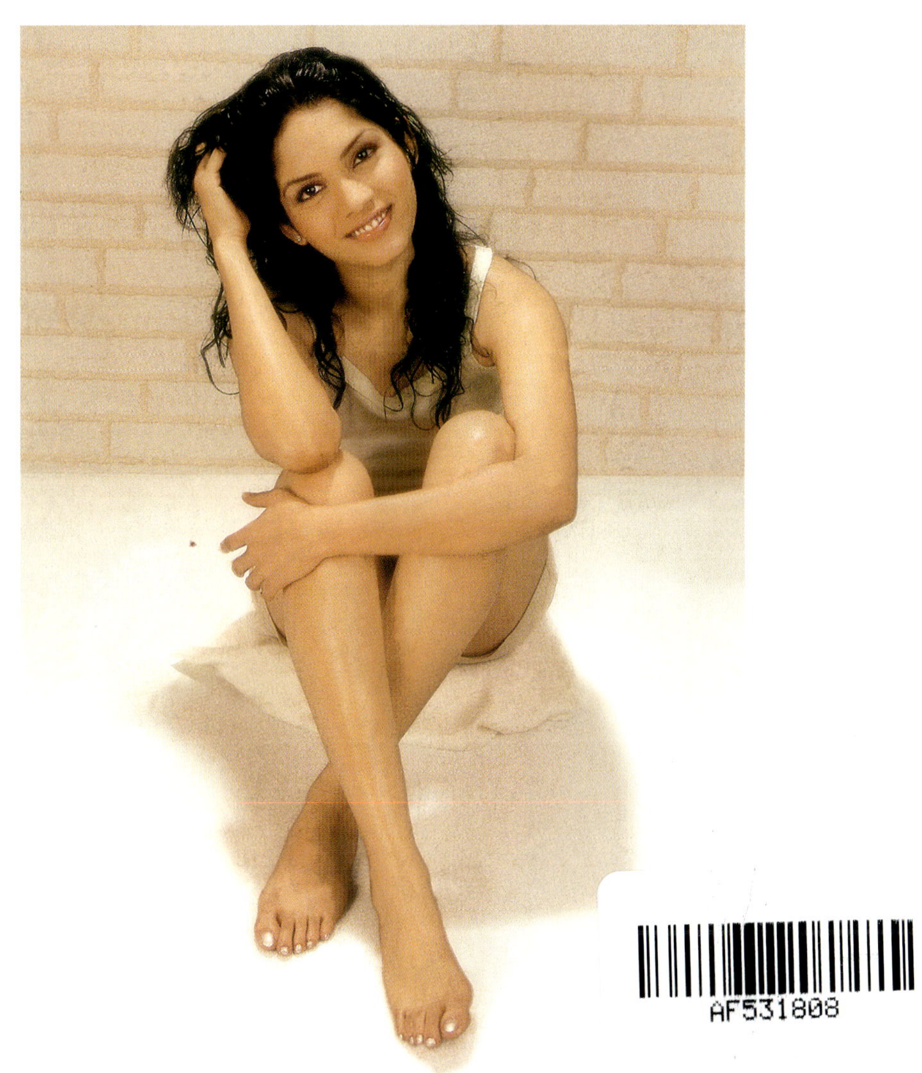

Ambika Manchanda

NATURALLY BEAUTIFUL

The Complete Beauty Book

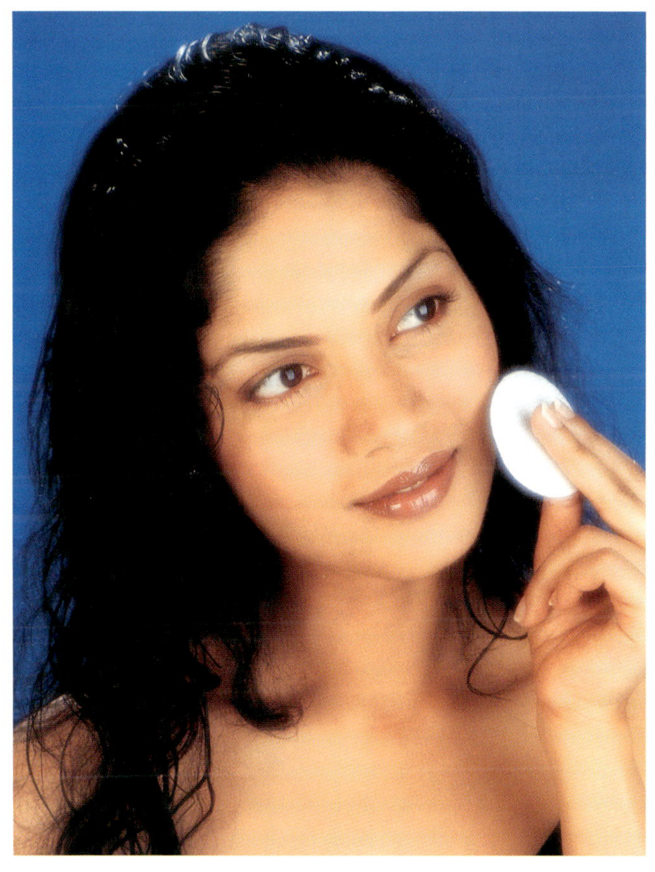

Rupa . Co

To my brother, Patanjali
and my father-in-law, Kailash

Sometimes you love because of circumstances.
And sometimes you love because of situations.
Sometimes you love no matter what.
And that is the best love there is.

First Published 2004
Second Impression 2010

Published by
Rupa Publications India Pvt. Ltd.
7/16, Ansari Road, Daryaganj,
New Delhi 110 002

Sales Centres:

Allahabad Bengaluru Chandigarh Chennai
Hyderabad Jaipur Kathmandu Kolkata
Mumbai

ISBN 81-291-0542-X

Cover, book design, concept and styling: Peali Dutta Gupta
Typeset in 10.5 pts. Photina MT by
The Studio, New Delhi 110 070

Printed in India by
Nutech Photolithographers
B-240, Okhla Industrial Area, Phase-I,
New Delhi 110 020, India

Contents

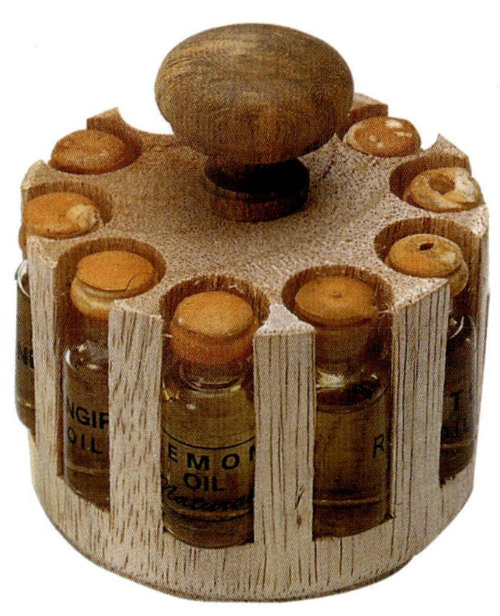

Foreword

Beauty is not the special shape of the eyebrows, the length of the hair, a tiny waist or dainty feet. It is more a way of expressing yourself, enhancing your physical assets and improving upon your drawbacks. Beauty is different things to different people. As the world changes, so do beauty concepts. How did black suddenly become beautiful? And lately, how is it that Indian women have taken all the top honours at the world beauty scene? Suddenly the world has woken up to the fact that beauty is not about looks, or colour, or about how to make up your face. It is much more than that. Its about being comfortable with one's own body. Its about health and vitality. And most of all, its about the knowledge that I am beautiful, because I feel beautiful inside.

Being beautiful is all about lifestyle. Not the way society columns depict wannabes. Its about doing the right things, eating the right foods, and having a fitness and beauty regimen. To do the right things, one has to know what to do. This book takes a major step in that direction. It tells you how you too can be beautiful, with simple and effective directions. The remedies could well take you back on a nostalgia trip. We go back to nature and its bounty. It's a fresh look at grandma's recipes, and the kitchen. A plethora of beauty aids and treatments; easy to make and simple to use. And the results? Wait and see.

Oriental women from China and India as well as those from ancient Egypt were superbly skilled in the art of repairing the ravages of time. They made lavish use of flowers, herbs and resins for making applications and potions that made their skin glow. The ancient art of make-up, face care, and beautifying the body were far more elaborate and advanced than today.

Shringar, or adornment, was considered almost a ritual for a bride. Traditionally and even today, at Hindu marriages the bride receives a beauty box from her husband. Today, synthetic mass manufactured vanity cases have replaced the ancient, adorably carved wooden chests or metal cases, once used by brides. Even the contents are mass products: a cream, a lipstick, a powder, and eyeliner and so on...as much as the purse permits. But in ancient times, the beauty box itself was a work of art. Much care was put into it and it was filled with all possible items for a woman's personal adornment. Glass or carved bottles of attar (extracts or perfumes) of roses, jasmine, mogra and many other flowers, containers of kohl for the eyes, others even more intricately carved or shaped containing abeer (power) or missi (a herb) to redden the lips were lovingly put into the make-up chest.

Today women all over the world are using henna to disguise white hair and turn it to a reddish brown shade. In ancient times henna has been used not only to enliven the hair but also to adorn the palms of the hands and feet and even colour the nails.

Teenagers today eagerly buy the latest anti-acne and antipimple creams at exorbitant prices, little realising that the cure for these ills exists in their own kitchens! Women in India have used sandalwood for centuries for this very purpose. It has strong antiseptic qualities and softens the skin. Similarly, women in most eastern countries have used "chikni mitti" or Fuller's earth, mixed with rose water. This is also popularly known as "Cleopatra's Pack" in the west. It helps to tighten the skin, and is the basis on which facemasks are marketed.

Women in ancient times were very particular about removing unwanted hair. Thus ash from incense sticks was used to get rid of them. Lemon juice and sugar mix was also used regularly for this purpose. Today, women go to beauty parlours for "waxing". Nothing changes. The future goes way back. Centuries back.

Women in India have always used herbs, fruits and flowers to beautify themselves, to adorn and enhance their good points. We do indeed have a wealth of knowledge as far as herbal and natural beauty aids are concerned. In fact beauty and make-up ritual in ancient times was more elaborate and state of the art than even today.

Exquisitely designed boxes and containers were used to store beauty aids. Historic evidence reveals that there was an intense desire for personal culture and body care. For instance, hair-drying pins of metal with intricately carved bases having devices for creating rhythmic sounds were used while drying the hair. These were very popular in South India. Among other objects of ancient toiletry articles, one can find slender bottles carved with tiny mirrors. Kankavatis were containers for a certain red pigment, used as bindis to mark the forehead.These containers had different forms like peacocks, musical instruments, elephants, swans, or mango.

Even the foot scrubbers found among ancient pieces were imaginatively made. These artefacts had a hollow shape and were fitted with tiny metal balls that made a rhythmic sound when used. Some other exquisitely shaped were containers for Missi, a herb to redden the lips; others contained different dyes to adorn the forehead. Carved boxes containing Abeer were also included. Abeer is a powder made from sandalwood, aloe, rose petals and a few grains of civet. These were powdered in a mortar to a very fine power.

Thus the ancient art of makeup and adornment finds no comparison today. In this jet age of instant cures, we look backwards to the glorious days when it was difficult to find an ordinary face, when women made it a point to look extraordinary.

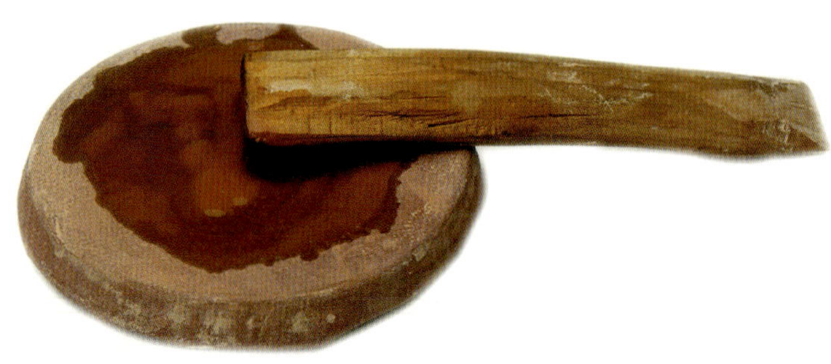

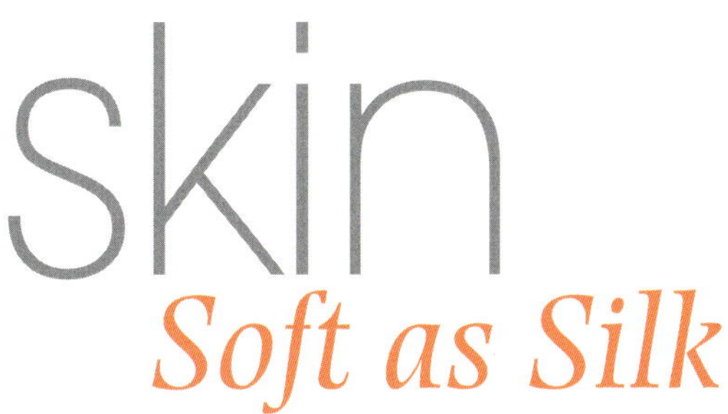

Soft as Silk

As soft as silk, as smooth as alabaster (marble), as fresh as a rose petal—poets and writers have gone into raptures while describing a woman's skin. Historically, the Egyptians were perhaps the first people who perfected the art of cosmetics and beautification techniques for the face, hair and the body. In fact they apparently went to great lengths to do so. The women improved their appearances by using a vast variety of cosmetics. The British Museum in London displays a beauty box dated 1400 BC, belonging to Queen Thuthu. The contents are fascinating. It contains pumice stones to remove rough skin, eye pencils of wood and ivory, with which probably kohl was applied, a bronze shallow dish used perhaps to mix ingredients for shading the eyes and several bottles of beauty potions.

Oriental women were known for their magical ability to deal with all beauty problems. It is only in the rush and run routine of the 20th century, that people have lost the art of looking beautiful. Today, most women go out and work. Obviously dust, pollution and a tension-ridden life can play havoc with your skin. Thus women end up using covering-up techniques by using make-up to hide their blemishes rather than using ancient and time tested methods to retain and enhance beauty. It's again a question of 'looking' beautiful, as against being naturally beautiful. This has certainly taken a heavy toll. Realisation has now dawned about the harmful effects of chemicals, and people are again going back to the basics: back to nature. Beauty lies there.

Now we turn back the pages of history and look and seek cosmetic cures from natural ingredients like fruits, flowers, and vegetables and herbs, along with different types of salts and soils, mud and earth. Granny's wisdom is evident in finding the right answers to all problems of beauty. A little knowledge, and a little time spent upon yourself can certainly help you to preserve God's gift of natural beauty.

To enhance your skin you need to understand your skin type and how to get the best from it. Your skin maxim should be minimum maintenance from natural resources. It should be improvement, rather than mere cover-up techniques.

Indeed, beautiful skin feels like soft, creamy, smooth silk. The colour matters little. Be it black, brown, or yellow or tan or white. Its beauty lies in its freshness, its softness and its smooth as silk looks. A good skin is a healthy skin. This shows that you care about yourself. The skin protects the body, keeps it at an even temperature. While poets have described it as a delicate part of our body, it's the skin that takes a batterings of a lifetime of wear and tear and gets the feel of leather. If you want to avoid this, then you must ensure a regular care regime for the skin.

To maintain the skin in a good condition, it needs to be constantly cleaned and cleared of dead cells that cause the pores to become blocked with dirt, pollution and sweat. The skin also needs to be constantly rejuvenated. Oxidation due to pollution, the sun's ultra violet rays; all contribute to wear and tear of the skin, blocking its pores and causing a host of other problems as well. Greasy skin, pimples, blackheads, roughened texture are all the results of neglect. Diet too plays an important role in determining the health of your skin.

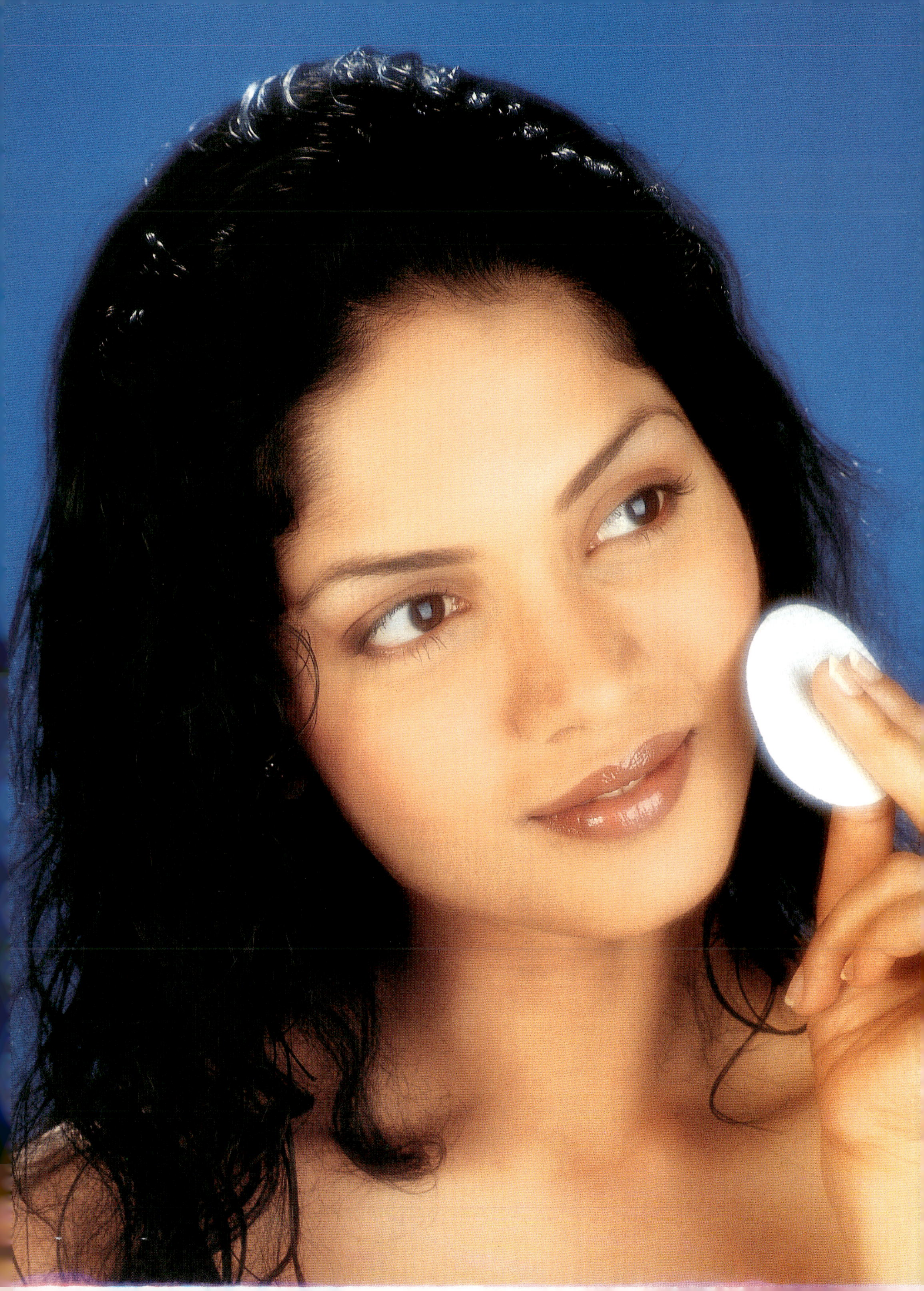

Skin Types

Basically there are three types of skin textures: normal, oily and dry. Some people have a dry skin in certain areas and an oily or normal skin in other areas. This is termed as a combination skin type.

NORMAL : This type of skin is neither too oily, nor too dry. It is not oversensitive to wind, harsh sunlight, or cold. It does not have open pores, lines or acne. It has a smooth texture. It poses little problems unless it has been neglected or abused.

OILY : Generally people develop an oily skin in their teens. Overproduction of oil by the sebaceous glands leads to an oily skin. People who have an oily skin should avoid oily food, starches and sugar. They need a rigid skin care regime and should remove every trace of make-up every night before going to bed. While bathing, mild exfoliates should be used.

DRY : Normally associated with ageing, some people have a naturally dry skin. In this case too, the right nourishment can work wonders. Along with this you need to have a moisturising routine.

Thus we see that all types of skin require care. The bath time is best for an overall skin caring routine. Bath time should not be a mere spartan exercise of cleansing the body. It should also be a time to revitalize your body and skin. True, in today's rush and run lifestyle, a morning bath can at most be a quick cleansing routine that 'wakes' you up for the day ahead. However, you could devote some extra time at night before going to bed when you bathe again. Also, a weekly, leisurely, rejuvenating bath should become a routine. This is when you could attend to your skin, and deal with any problem.

Tiny body pimples caused by over secretion of the sebaceous glands are a result of poor circulation. Use a loofah or coarse mitt to scrub these away and renew your skin. A pumice stone should be used for your heels and other rough areas like elbows and knees. Normal wrinkling of the skin can be attended to while bathing. Rub some moisturizing cream or lotion before the bath. Massage well, and then wash away.

You would be surprised to know that your kitchen is a magical box that has all the ingredients to make you beautiful. Expensive creams and lotions are certainly not the answer to your beauty problems. Flowers, fruits, vegetables and other natural things can provide the answers to a lot of skincare problems. So let's start with something really exciting and unusual...but very simple.

Floral Baths

The Romans, Egyptians and oriental women were known to have very fastidious beauty and bathing routines. For them, bathing was a major social event. They also promoted the healing powers of warm water to which various herbs, salts and flowers were added, thus ensuring health-giving qualities to their baths.

MIXED HERBS AND LEAF BATH : Take a handful of bay leaves, rosemary and chamomile leaves. Put all these together in a piece of muslin. Tie it tight and soak this bundle in your bathtub or water bucket in slightly warm water for half an hour. The fragrance permeates into the water. Remove the bundle of muslin and gently rub it all over your body and then bathe with the fragrant water. This bath is most relaxing and helps tone up the body.

FLORAL BATH : Chamomile flowers, rose petals or fragrant tube roses, even agrimony, wrapped in a muslin cloth or bag, soaked in water would have the same toning and smoothening effect upon your skin.

MILK BATH : A traditional elaborate bath that literally 'feeds' your skin! Considered to be the very height of luxury, it was used by Nero's wife, Poppaea, and has since been a favourite over the years. Poppaea bathed in donkey's milk and water. Several innovations have been introduced to make this a fascinating bath regime. It's easily made at home.

Take Half Litre Milk. To this add 2 tablespoons of honey. Add strained chamomile juice or the juice of crushed rose petals obtained by infusing them in water. Mix all these and pour the mixture into warm bath water. Soak yourself in the bathtub, or keep pouring slowly over your body, rubbing all over. Be leisurely about this. After the milk and flower water has been used up. You could bathe with normal cold water.

BATH FOR DRY SKIN : Take 200 ml. of glycerin, and add to this 200 ml. of rose water. Pour this in a bottle. Smear this all over your body and beginning at the neck, start rubbing it in gently as you go downwards, to your arms, torso, legs and back. Continuously massage the mixture into your skin, nourishing it. Once the solution is absorbed into the skin take a normal bath using a glycerin-based soap.

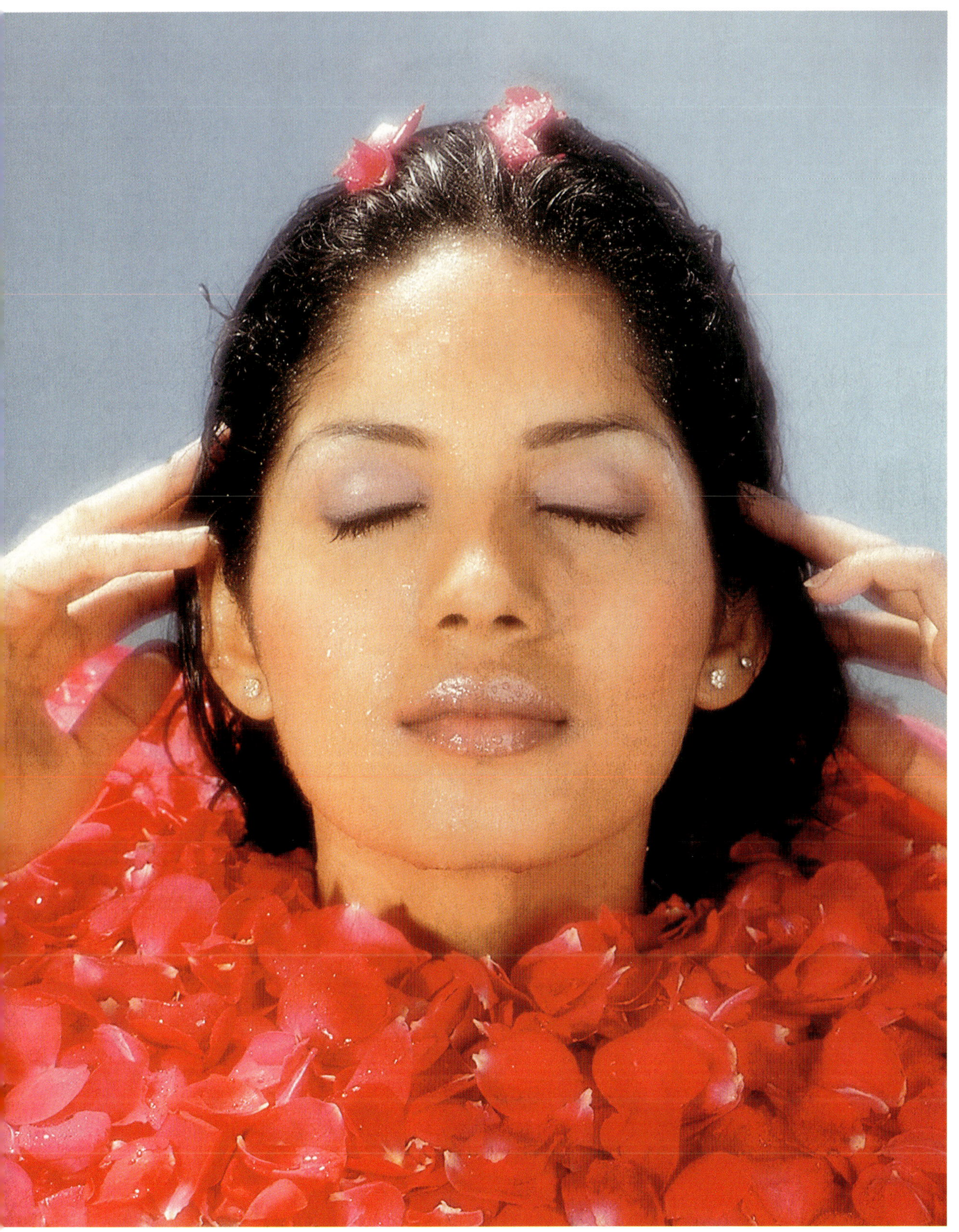

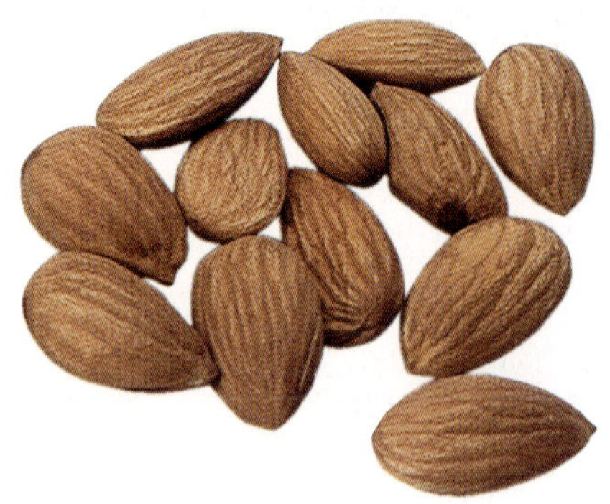

ALMOND BATH : This is also an ideal solution for people with a dry skin. It should be used especially during severe winters when even normal and oily skins tend to dry up. You should use this treatment instead of soap. Take a piece of muslin, crush a few almonds and tie them in it. Wet your body; rub this almond bag all over your body vigorously. Keep adding a little water and continue scrubbing. This immediately exfoliates without damaging your skin and at the same time it nourishes the skin with its natural oils.

VINEGAR BATH : Those with an oily skin problem should definitely try this. Take a mug of water and add to it a little malt vinegar. Mix well and massage your body with this diluted vinegar water. Take a bath with cold water and feel the difference.

MILK AND EGG BATH : Wrinkling skin? Do not fret. Try out this simple magical formula. Take a cup of cold milk. Take the white of one egg and beat it up until it stiffens. Add the cold milk and fold it gently into the egg. Use this paste all over beginning at the neck, down the arms, torso and legs. Leave it on for five minutes. It dries very quickly. Then bathe with a mild soap. It leaves the skin looking taut and supple.

CUCUMBER AND YOGURT BATH : Take one cucumber. Peel it and chop it into small pieces. Take half cup of curd and add to it the chopped cucumber pieces. Then run it through a blender to form a thick paste. Apply this paste all over the face, neck and body before a bath. Leave it on for 7-10 minutes. Rub vigorously and then bathe with a mild soap. This is a very nourishing and cooling bath routine and goes down well in the hot summer months.

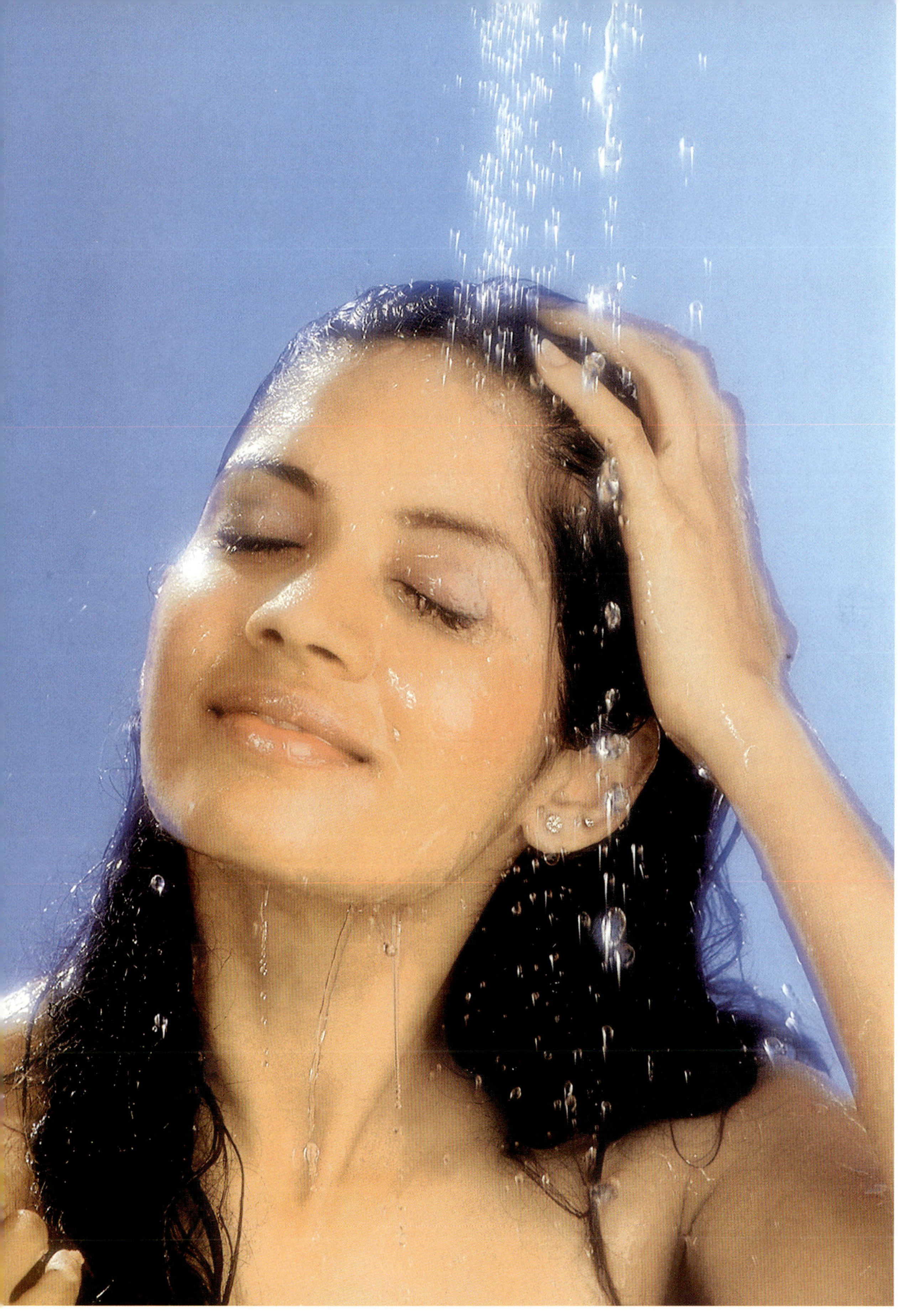

Scrubs

Dead skin cells, jaded skin and tanning can effectively be got rid off by using exfoliating scrubs to remove dead cells. However, do not exfoliate everyday. If your skin is oily, it needs to be done maybe once a week. For those with dry skins exfoliating twice a month is sufficient. You can easily make some homemade scrubs that can be as effective. Try them.

ORANGE AND LEMON PEEL SCRUB : Do not throw away orange and lime, or lemon peels. Dry them out thoroughly till they are brittle. While drying them, keep them away from sunlight. Powder them and keep them in a jar. Take two tablespoons of the dried peel power, two tablespoons of wheat bran or porridge grains. Add to this half tablespoon of honey and a little milk to make a coarse paste. Before a bath, rub this all over your neck, arms, body and legs. Use rough circular motions as you go along. This will help to exfoliate dead skin. Then bathe normally. It's a wonderful scrub and so easy to make and the effects are immediately visible. Leaves you feeling squeaky-clean.

CHICKPEA POWDER SCRUB : If your skin is oily this is the ideal homemade scrub. Take 4 tablespoons of chickpea powder. Add to this, half tablespoons of turmeric power, a few drops of rose water and milk to make a thick paste. Rub it all over the body. When the paste dries and starts caking, again use rough circular motions to exfoliate. People with dry skin can also use this scrub after substituting milk with full cream.

OATS : Take half a litre of buttermilk or half a litre of beaten curds. Take half a cupful of oats that have been coarsely ground or are in thick powdered form. Add to the curd or butter milk. Mix well. Pour in a container and refrigerater for 2 hours. Apply this thick paste all over the body starting from the neck downwards, to the arms, torso and legs. Leave it on for 20 minutes. Rinse off with warm water containing lemon juice. This scrub reduces pores and cleans up the skin.

TOMATO WRAP : Take 4 tomatoes. Chop them finely. Puree them. Soak some rice for 30 minutes and then grind it coarsely. Add this to the pureed tomatoes. Apply all over and leave it on for about 20 minutes. Bathe with warm water. A good scrub for people with oily skins.

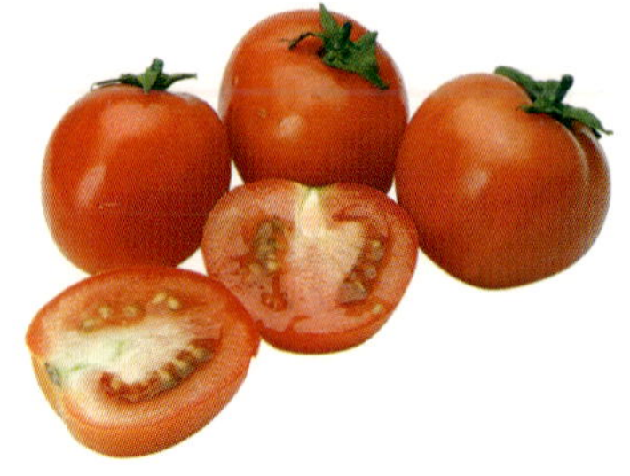

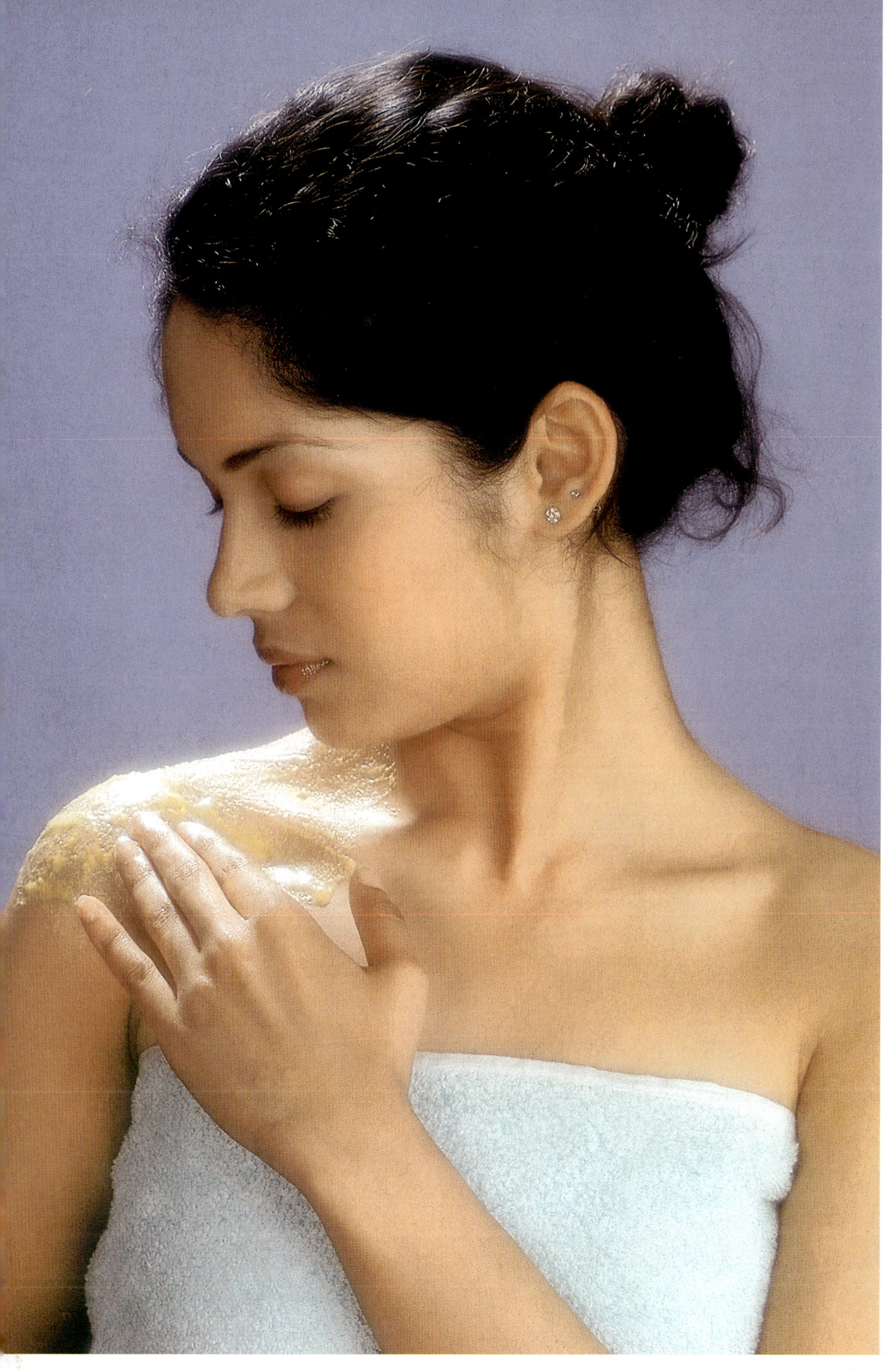

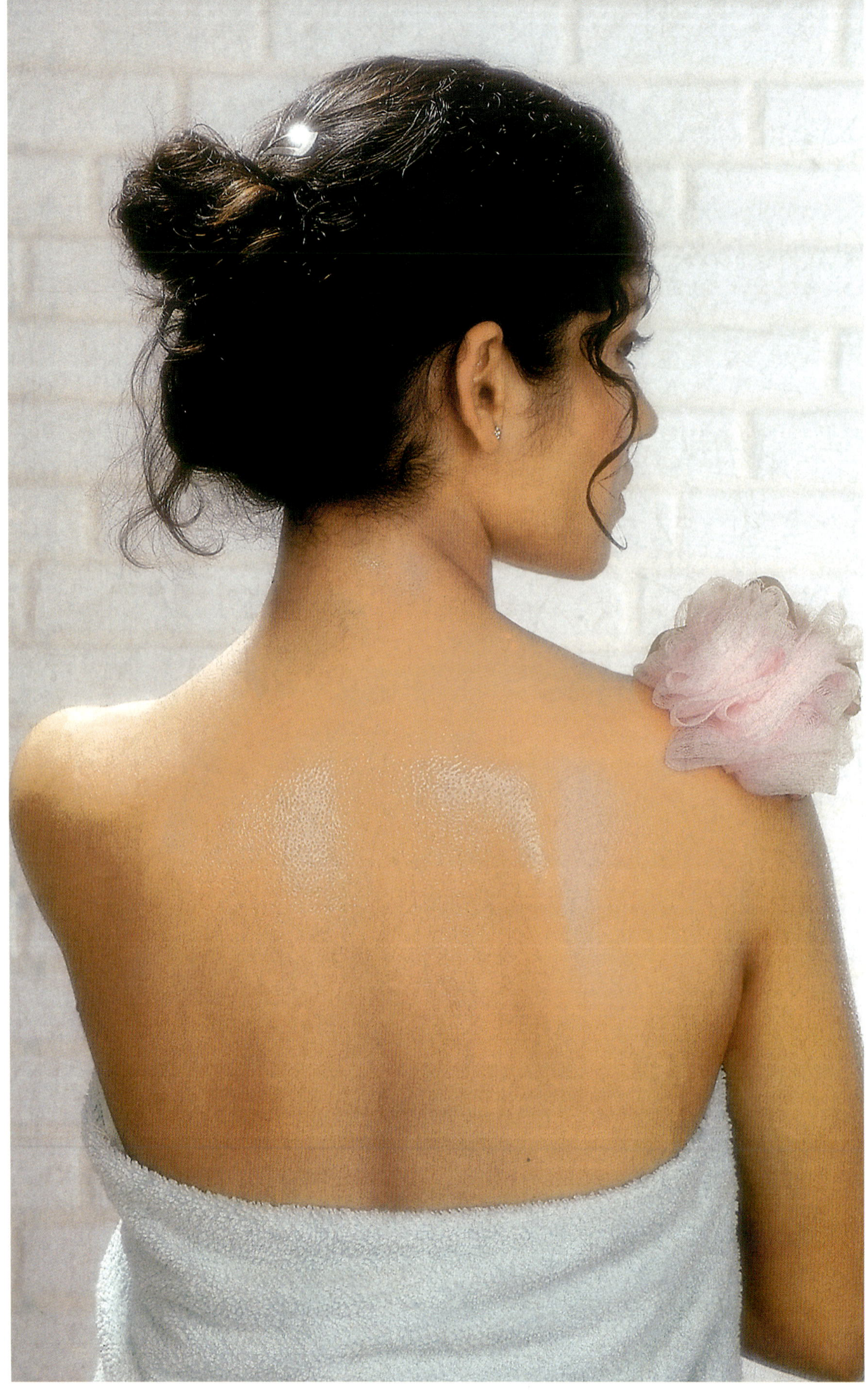

Bathing Routines

You can have different types of bathing routines to suit the needs of your skin. The body loses a fair amount of natural oils after a bath. You constantly need to replenish them.

SAFFRON : Take half cup olive oil and half cup almond oil. Add to it a pinch of saffron. Mix them together and pour in a small pan with a handle. Take a large container with water and put it to boil. Hold the small pan over the container and steam it well, constantly stirring the mixture till the oils obtain a rich yellow colour. Remove and cool. Pour the oils into a bottle and keep for further use. Use this after a bath. Gently massage all over the body, neck downwards. Keep massaging till the skin completely absorbs the oils. It is very soothing, nourishing for the skin and the saffron gives a heady perfume.

SANDALWOOD OIL : Take a cupful of coconut oil, and one teaspoon of sandalwood oil. Mix well; pour into a jar to keep for use. Massage well into the body after a bath. Tones up the skin and gives a very luxurious and vitalizing feeling.

ROSEWATER AND GLYCERIN : Take half a cup of glycerin. Add to this 250 ml of rose water. Stir well and pour into a bottle to keep for use. Massage all over your body after a bath. This is one of the mildest and most nourishing of skin conditioners.

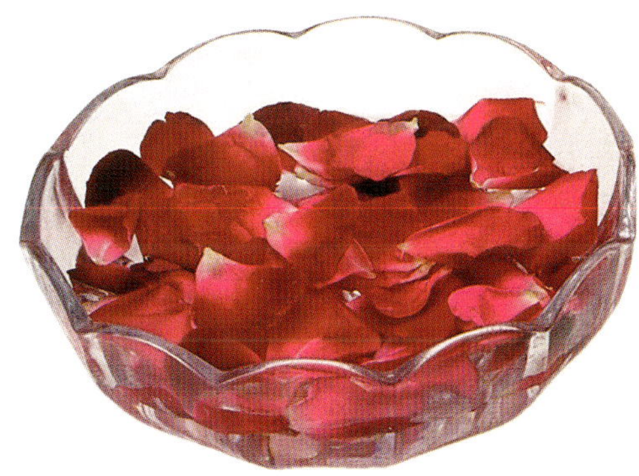

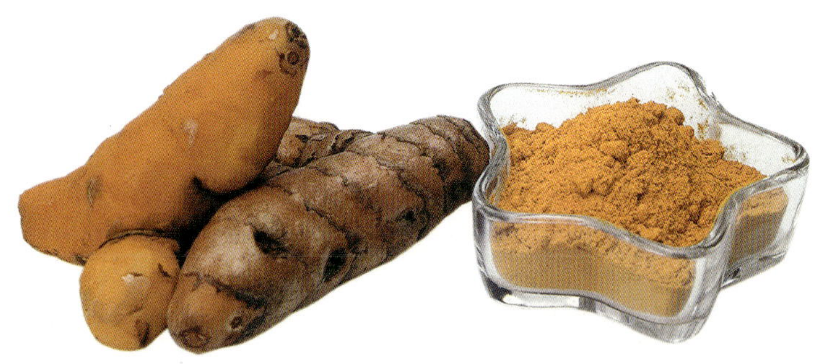

Skin Problems

Kitchen disasters and neglect can cause burns, bruises and even chilblains. These are negging problems which have surprisingly simple cures.

Burns

YOUR SKIN DOES NEED PAMPERING. Skincare should be a routine rather than management by crisis. It needs to be a good habit and not an exception before any occasion. Pampering your skin with oils, lotions, masks and scrubs is certainly not the end. You need to have a balanced diet too. Foods like salads, fruits and vegetables, coupled with Vitamin A enriched foods are good for your skin. Curds, honey and tons of water give way to a fresh and youthful skin.

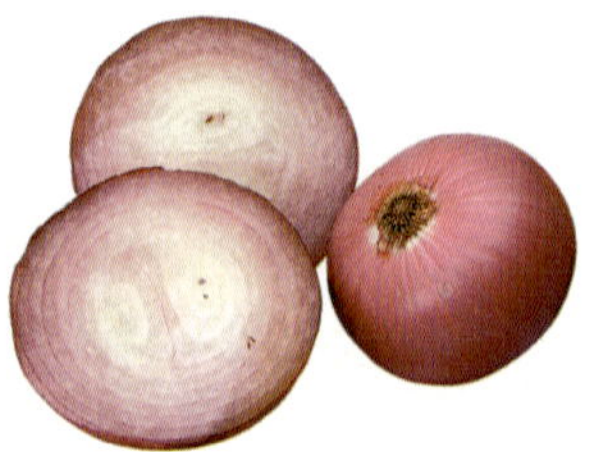

ONIONS : Most minor burns at home occur in the kitchen by touching hot stoves, ovens, food containers and hot irons. These are usually superficial in nature and can be treated at home. The key is to act quickly and maintain presence of mind and soothe the skin. Run cold water over the burn for 5 minutes. Take a raw onion, slice it and rub the cut surface of the onion over the burn area. It relieves the pain and reduces the inflammation.

TURMERIC : This has tremendous curative power. Use a paste of turmeric and curd on the burn immediately. Apply the paste gently. Leave it on. Wash off and leave the skin to dry completely. Repeat after some time.

POTATOES : Immediately slice a raw potato and place the raw slices over the burn and bandage lightly. Keep the bandage on for about 20-30 minutes. This immediately gives a cooling effect and also helps in removal of scars. Alternatively you could boil and mash the potatoes and apply them as a pack over the burnt area. This will help in lightening the scars and over time will remove them.

CABBAGE : A similar cabbage leaf poultice also helps.

CAMPHOR AND COCONUT OIL : If the burn has left scars then try this. Crush 2 tablets of camphor and add to it 250 ml of coconut oil. Mix well till the camphor dissolves in the oil. Pour the oil into a jar. Apply regularly over the burn scar. It helps to lighten and remove the scar.

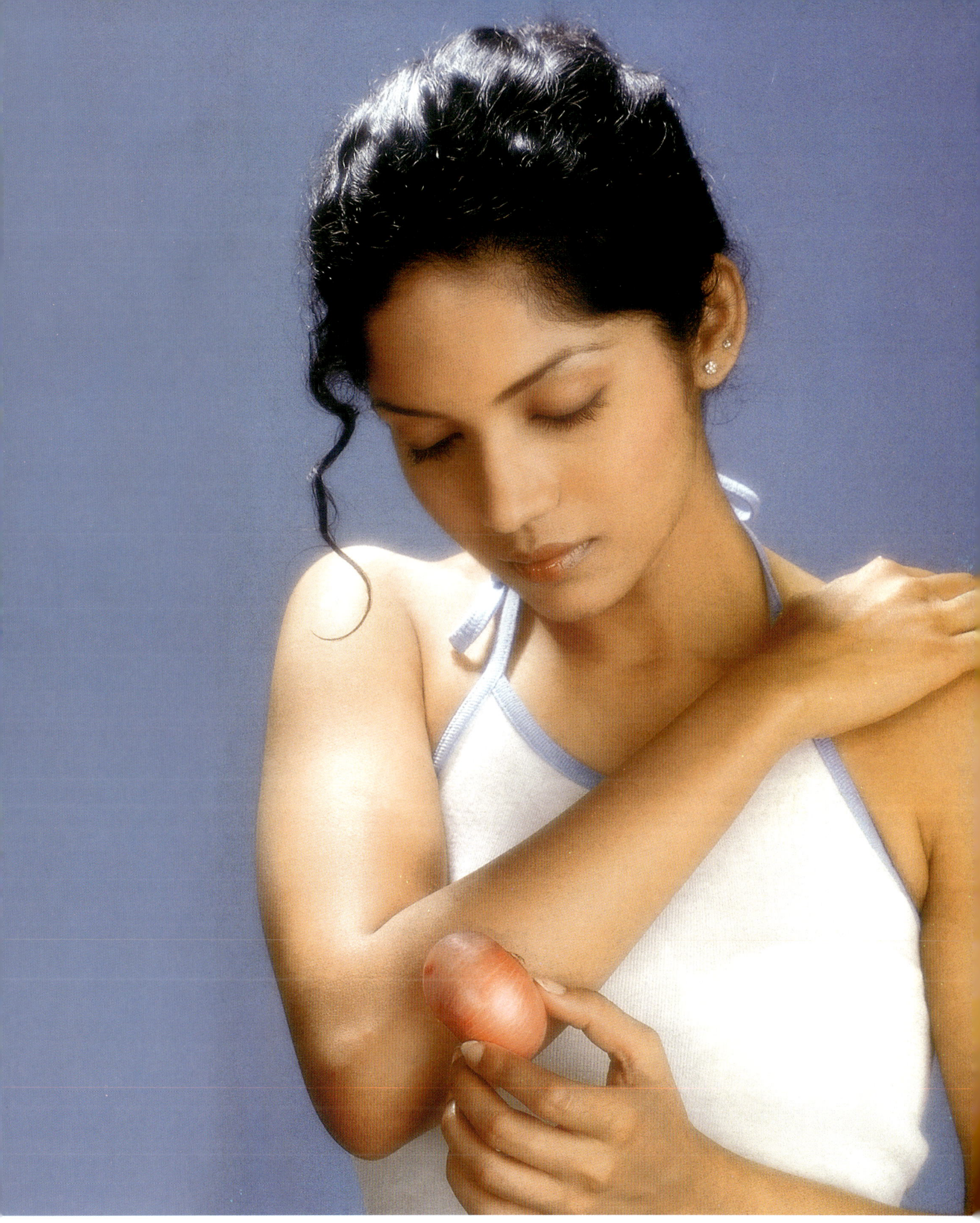

ALOE VERA : A very useful plant. It has multifarious uses in skincare problems. Should be kept accessible. Just break off a leaf and squeeze the moisture on the brim. Soothes immediately. These days Aloe Vera gel is easily available at all chemists and beautician's shop too as it is a very popular skin hydrant.

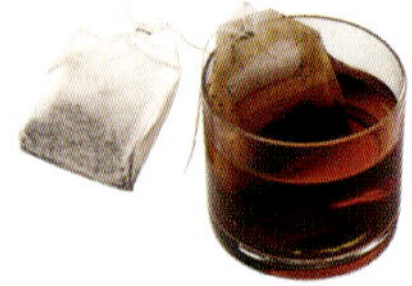

TEA : Use wet tea bags. Apply them over the burnt area and keep them moist till the pain is reduced. This prevents blistering.

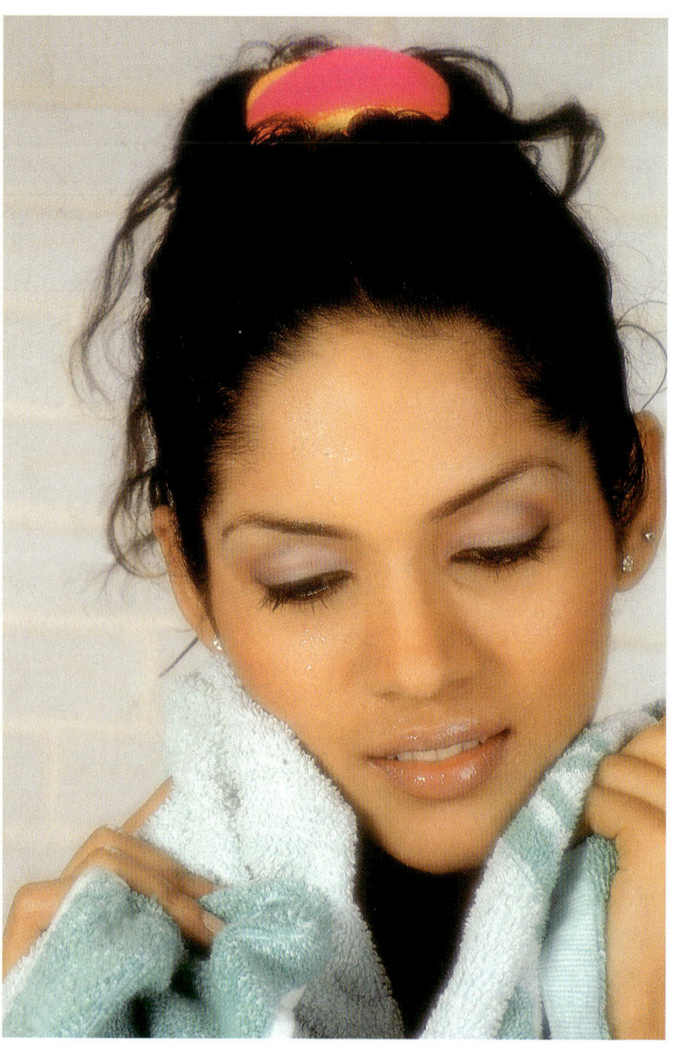

Perspiration

We all perspire. Some of us do so very profusely, while for others it is normal. There are 2 million sweat glands all over the body. You need to use deodorants and anti-perspirants after a bath, more so in summers. You could use sprays, talcum powders or lotions to keep you smelling fresh and appearing cool. A vast variety is available today. Choose these products to suit your skin type. People with oily skins should avoid roll-ons and cream deodorants. Instead, they should use dry sprays. However, light talcum powders are best. Use them after your bath; allow them to dry completely before putting on your clothes.

Chilblains

These itchy, reddish blue swellings occur in winter on fingers and toes. They occur due to cold that restricts blood circulation in the extremities. Here are a few simple home remedies for this problem.

ONION : If you suffer from chilblains use this remedy regularly during winter. Cut a raw onion. Use the cut edge all over the chilblains; let the juice soak into the skin. The severity of itching dies down almost instantly.

EGG AND HONEY : Taka a tablespoon of honey, a little glycerin, and one egg white, and add to this a little flour. Mix in to a paste. Apply all over the chilblains. Leave it on for 6-8 hours. Wash off. Cures you very quickly.

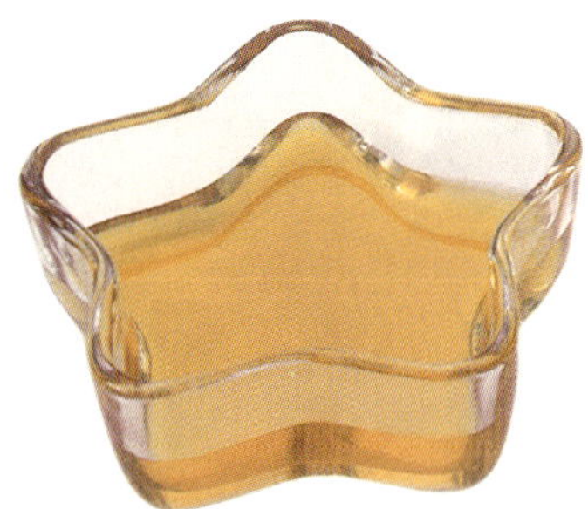

POTATO : Slice a potato. Sprinkle some salt on it. Rub it all over the chilblains. Helps to soothe the itching and redness.

Minor Cuts & Bruises

EASTER LILY : These belong to the same family as the garlic and onion. They have tremendous curative powers. They are rich in aromatic anti-microbial oils, which make them effective in curing minor cuts and bruises.

Take a handful of lily petals. Rinse in warm water. Chop finely. Cover them by rubbing alcohol and then set them aside for two weeks. Now crush these, strain the juice and pour it into a small bottle. Apply gently on cuts and wounds.

We thus see that knowledge of the use of plants, flowers, fruits and basic kitchen condiments and herbs can take care of most of our skin care problems. Above all, you need to be conscientious in the effort to keep a healthy skin.

Hands and Feet

Hands are the most used or rather the most abused part of our body. Yet, they have inspired poets to write poems on them. They are the most visible and vulnerable part of our body.

Hands and feet are constantly exposed and perform a zillion different tasks. Since they do not have any oil glands to protect them from within, they also dry up faster and tend to wrinkle and age faster. Our hands also pay a heavy price due to lack of care. We tend to overlook them and use them in lieu of tools, doing numerous chores. In fact, since they work the hardest, they need special care and pampering.

Our overworked and indispensable pair of hands are busy all the time, dusting, cleaning, cooking, scrubbing, washing, typing—in fact, they are seldom still; perhaps only when one sleeps. They do achieve incredible tasks and as a result face the maximum punishments or accidents. They get burnt while cooking, cut and bruised while chopping and scrubbing. They do need extra care and attention.

In fact, since they are so visible, they need to look their best all the time. You can camouflage your face with make-up but you cannot hide ugly, uncared for, misused hands. So, do spare a thought for these overworked hands.

Romantically, hands have figured in many a poet's literary expression, and delicate, 'rose-petal' hands have been considered to be a sign of a beautiful woman.

Constant exposure to the elements and harsh chemicals makes our hands dry faster. The nails too get discoloured, crack, chip, and become hard and brittle due to exposure to chemicals in detergents. Diet also affects the health of your nails. Lack of certain vitamins discolours the nails and makes them brittle. Thus, you have to be careful about your food intake to maintain a healthy pair of hands and beautiful almond shaped and pearly nails.

Some of the common problems that make hands harsh and nails brittle and hard have been tackled here. Useful tips and common cures by using natural products from the kitchen are listed to enable you to take good care of your hands and nails.

The key to a beautiful pair of hands is regular care and maintenance. Most of us ignore our hands and feet. It is absolutely important to establish a hand and foot care routine.

Start by washing your hands with a mild glycerin based soap. Next, exfoliate your hands with any good home made exfoliate. Now place your hands in warm water, to which olive oil and a mild soap has been added. Soak them in this water and scrub the nails using a soft nails brush. Remove and pat them dry.

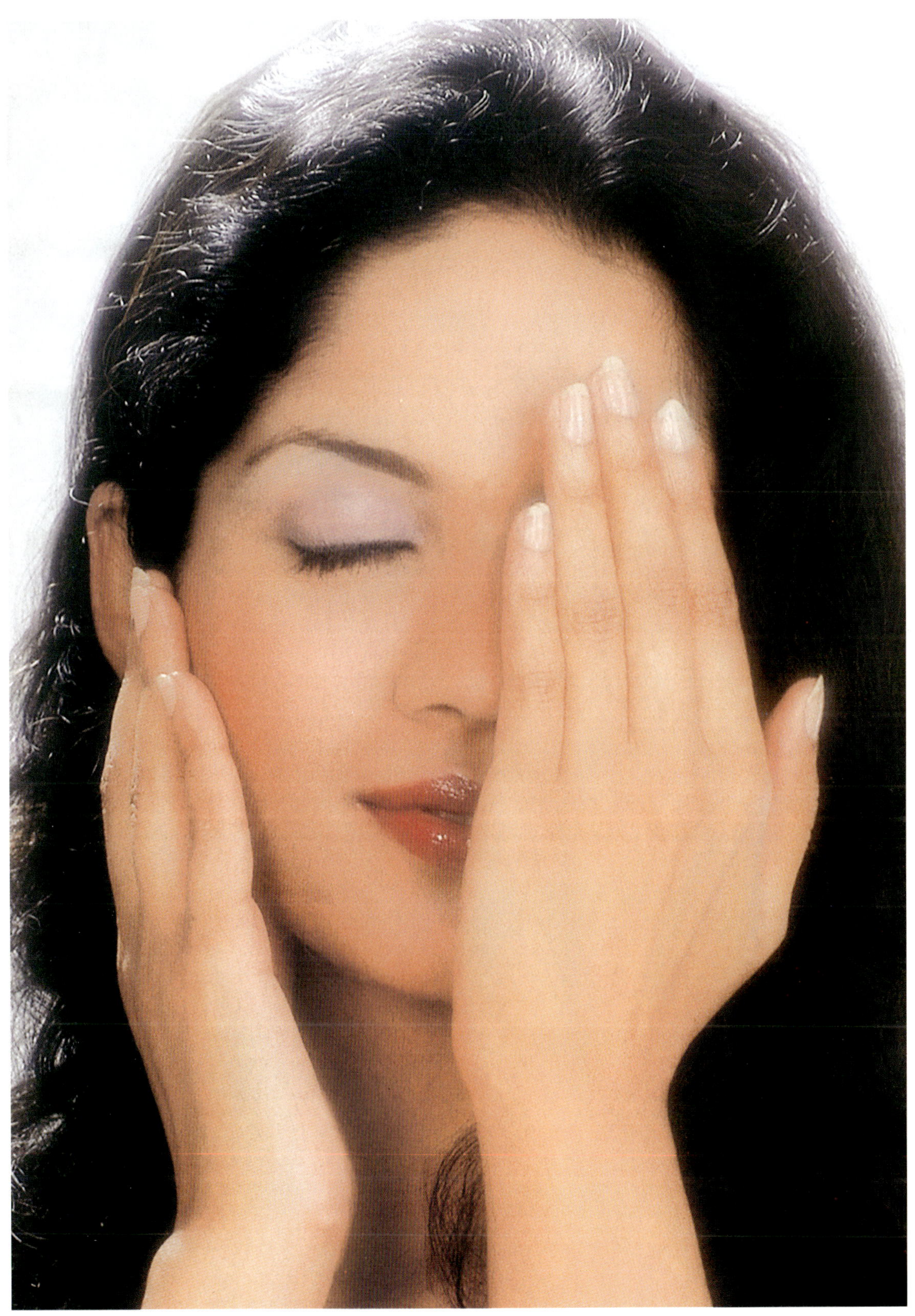

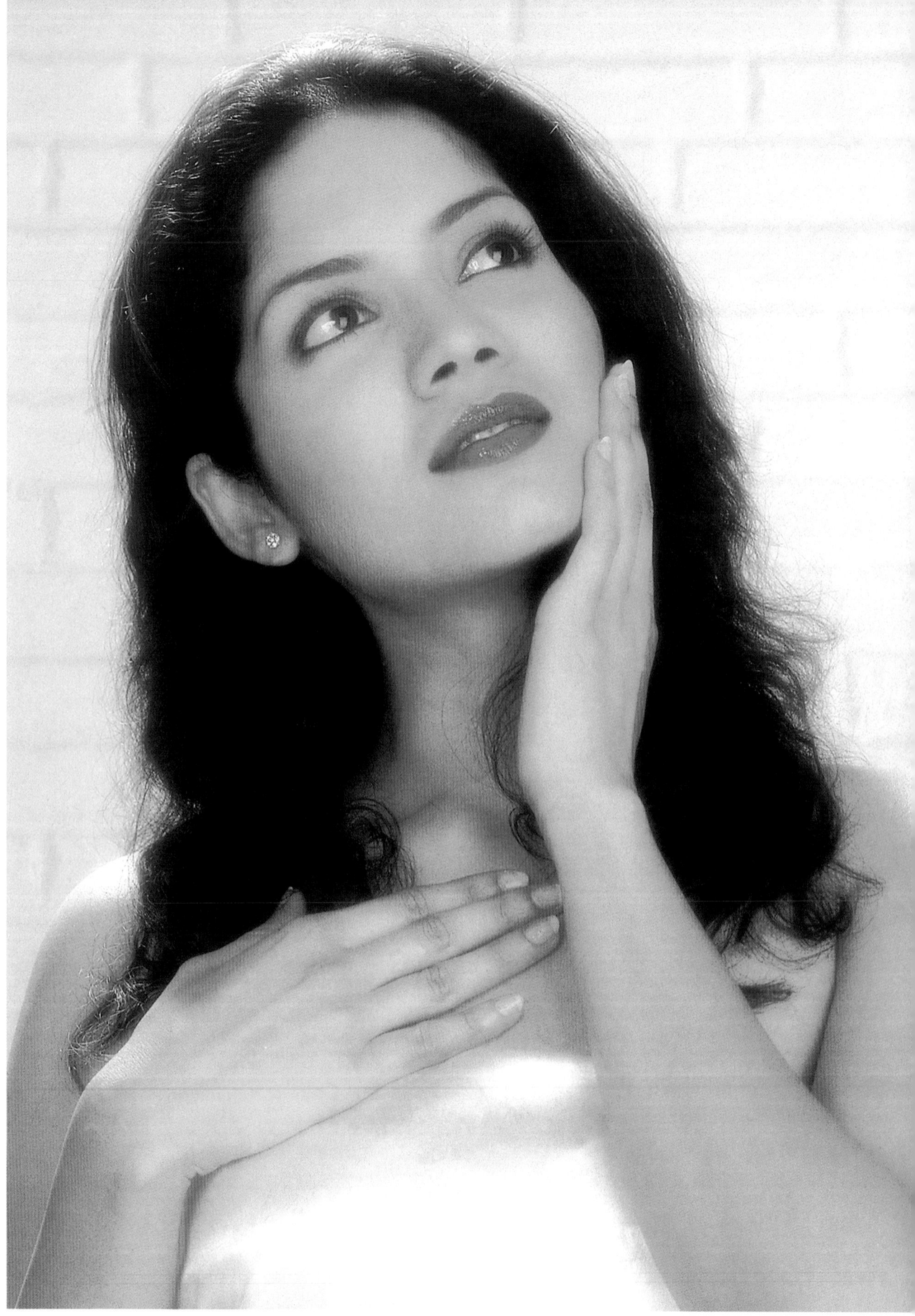

Take some warm olive oil or almond oil and massage into the hands. Keep massaging each finger. Start at the tips, go to the knuckles. When you moisturize or cream your hands, use firm swivelling motions with your forefinger and thumb to massage the oil or the lotion into each finger of the other hand. Rub oil or the moisturizer onto the knuckles and cuticles as well. This helps improve the circulation too.

While massaging, exercise your fingers. Pull each fingers. Close your first, open it. Repeat constantly. It lubricates your hands and gives them a soothing exercise.

Massage creams or moisturizers at least twice a day, once after a bath and once at bedtime. In winters the hands need to be moisturized more often.

Keep a cut lime near your working sink. Rub lime on your hands and nails before doing kitchen work. It helps to keep the nails from getting brittle.

Dip your hands in milk for 10 minutes everyday. Its helps in keeping them supple.

While doing household chores like washing, dusting or scrubbing, put on rubber gloves. This will prevent your hands from being exposed to harsh detergents and chemicals.

Just simple, precautionary measures like these would improve the look of your hands. There are some useful, easily available creams and lotions which would also enhance the beauty of your hands.

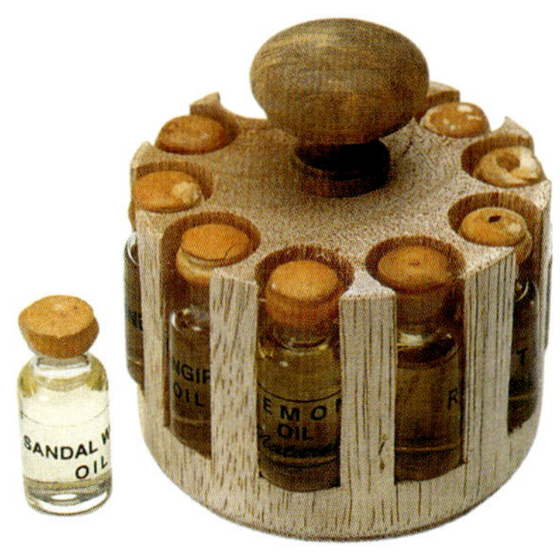

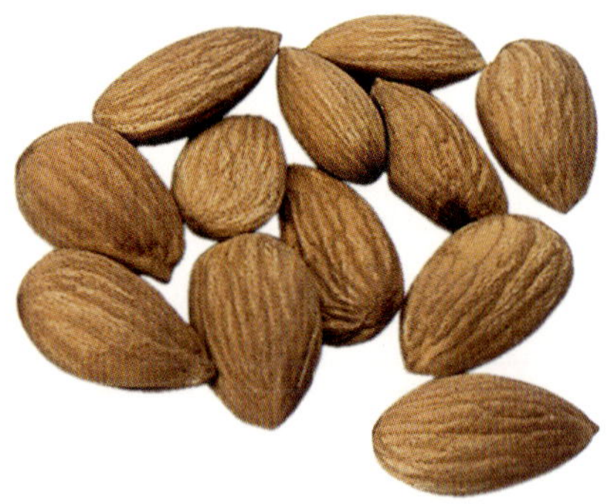

Hand Creams and Lotions

As mentioned earlier, there are three types of skin textures : normal, oily and dry. Each type therefore requires a different hand cream or lotion.

EGG AND ALMOND NOURISHER : In winter your hands need extra nourishment. Try this excellent nourishment for your hands—:

One egg, Two tablespoons of almond oil, One tablespoon rose water

Beat all the ingredients well. Take half teaspoon tincture benzoin, add drop by drop, mixing well. Apply this lotion on your hands. Leave it on for at least 2 hours. Wash off. An excellent luxury nourishment for the hands.

MILK : Warm 2 cups of milk and pour into a bowl. Add a teaspoonful of salt and stir. Soak hands in warm milk and salt solution. Keep massaging and rubbing around the knuckles and finger joints. Wash off after 10-15 minutes. This exfoliates and nourishes your hands.

ROSE PETAL HAND LOTION : 1/3 cup glycerin and 2/3 cup rose water. Combine both ingredients. Shake well and pour in a bottle. Store in a cool, dry place. Use several times a day to massage into your hands. Makes the hands soft. It is an ideal softener during winter months.

CURD : Take one cup of curd, and to it add a little lime juice. Beat it up and pour into a bowl. Dip your hands into it, all the time massaging and rubbing around the knuckles and finger joints. After 10 minutes wash off with plain water. This is excellent for sunburned hands or those that have been exposed to chemicals and detergents. It acts as a balm, and also lightens the tan on your hands.

BANANA AND HONEY CREAM: One banana, one teaspoon honey, juice of one lemon, one table spoon butter or margarine.

Mash the banana and add to it the honey, lime juice and butter. Blend well together and put it in a container. Apply well, massaging well with firm strokes into your hands. Leave on for 2 hours, then wash off. The hands become very soft and smooth.

HONEY AND ORANGE JUICE: Half cup orange juice, one tablespoon honey.

Mix well together, and then rub into your hands and nails. Leave it on for 10 minutes. Rinse off. This is an ideal solution for dry, rough and chapped hands.

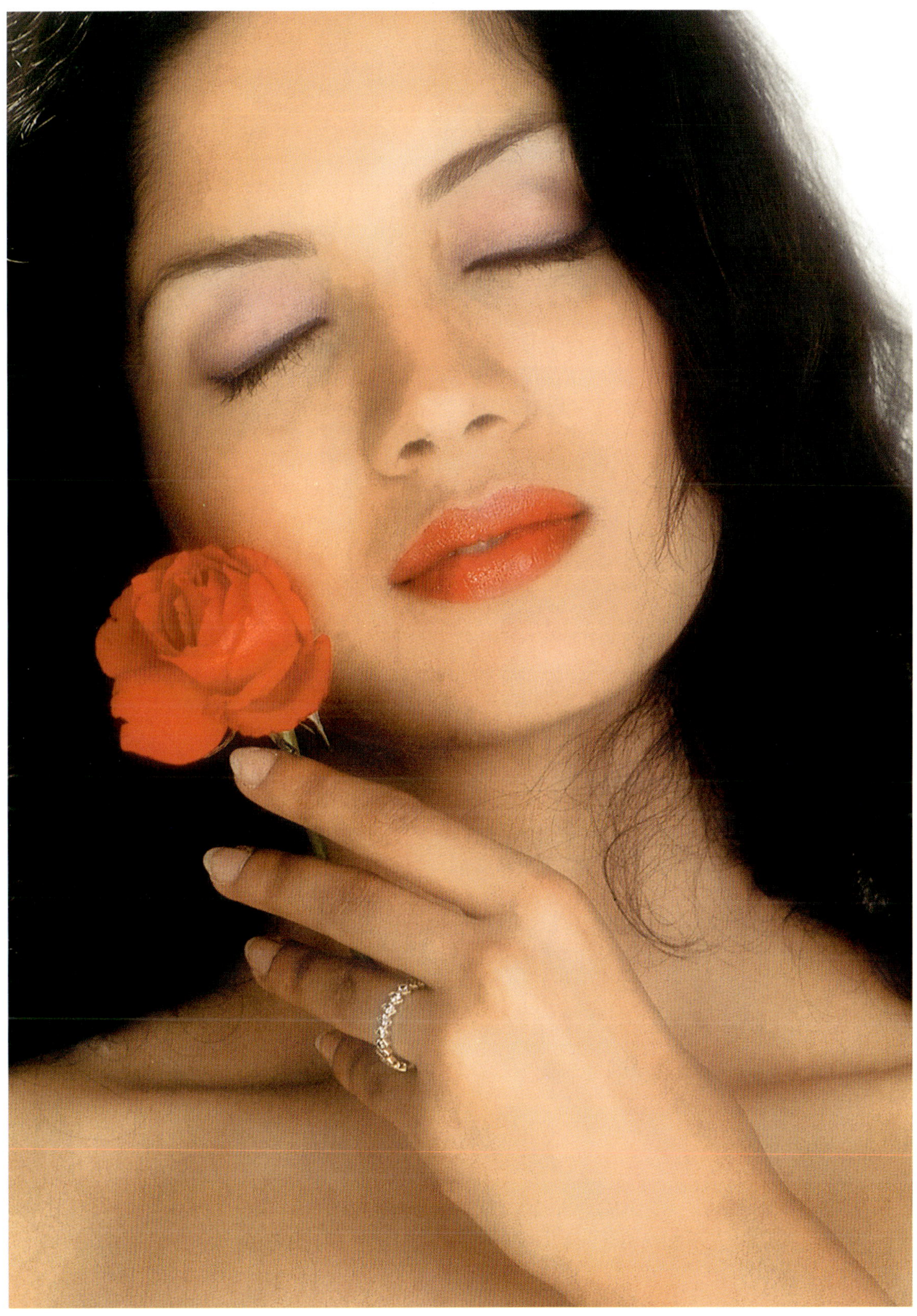

Dry Hands

Most of us have our pet peeves about our hands. Some have dry coarse hands; others have cold clammy hands. Some have soft thin delicate hands where the skin tears easily. A little knowledge would help you to overcome some of these problems. Apart from this, one is constantly exposed to minor cuts, burns and bruns and bruises in the kitchen or while doing chores. Here are some good tips to rectify these problems.

SUGAR AND OIL : Take 3 tablespoons of sugar, 2 tablespoons of oil (any oil, vegetable oils, olive oil or almond oil will do). Mix the sugar and oil, beat to a blended consistency. Rub into the hands. Keep rubbing for 5-7 minutes, then rinse well with warm water. The dead coarse skin is removed and the hands appear soft and clean.

SUGAR AND LIME : Take one tablespoon lemon juice, one tablespoon sugar, one tablespoon water. Lightly mix all these ingredients and rub all over the hands. Keep rubbing it in till it starts to dry. Rinse with water. Softens coarse hands.

HONEY LEMON JUICE AND OIL : Take one-teaspoon oil (any oil, vegetable oils, olive oil or almond oil will do), one teaspoon lemon juice, one tablespoon rose water. Mix well together. Rub over crusty elbows, knuckles and other hardened areas. Keep rubbing it in, then after 5-7 minutes rinse off. This not only nourishes the skin, but also keeps it soft.

LEMON JUICE AND BARELY POWDER : Take one tablespoon barley powder, one tablespoon lime juice.

In case barley powder is not available, boil barley for 10 minutes. Extract the juice and mix it with lime juice. Apply on the finger joints to get rid of dark circles. Rub well into the skin. Leave it to dry and then apply and rub again. After it has dried, then rinse off. Softens and whitens the knuckles.

POTATO JUICE : Take two potatoes, peel and grate them. Extract juice of these potatoes. Apply all over the hands, especially over the knuckles and finger joints. The potato juice can also be applied over scars left by wounds, cuts or burns. If used regularly, it helps to eliminate these scars and lightens dark areas around the knuckles and finger joints.

ONION JUICE : You can relieve minor kitchen burns on the hand just by rubbing a raw onion on the burn. Take an onion, cut it into half and rub on the burned area. It immediately reduces inflammation and relieves pain.

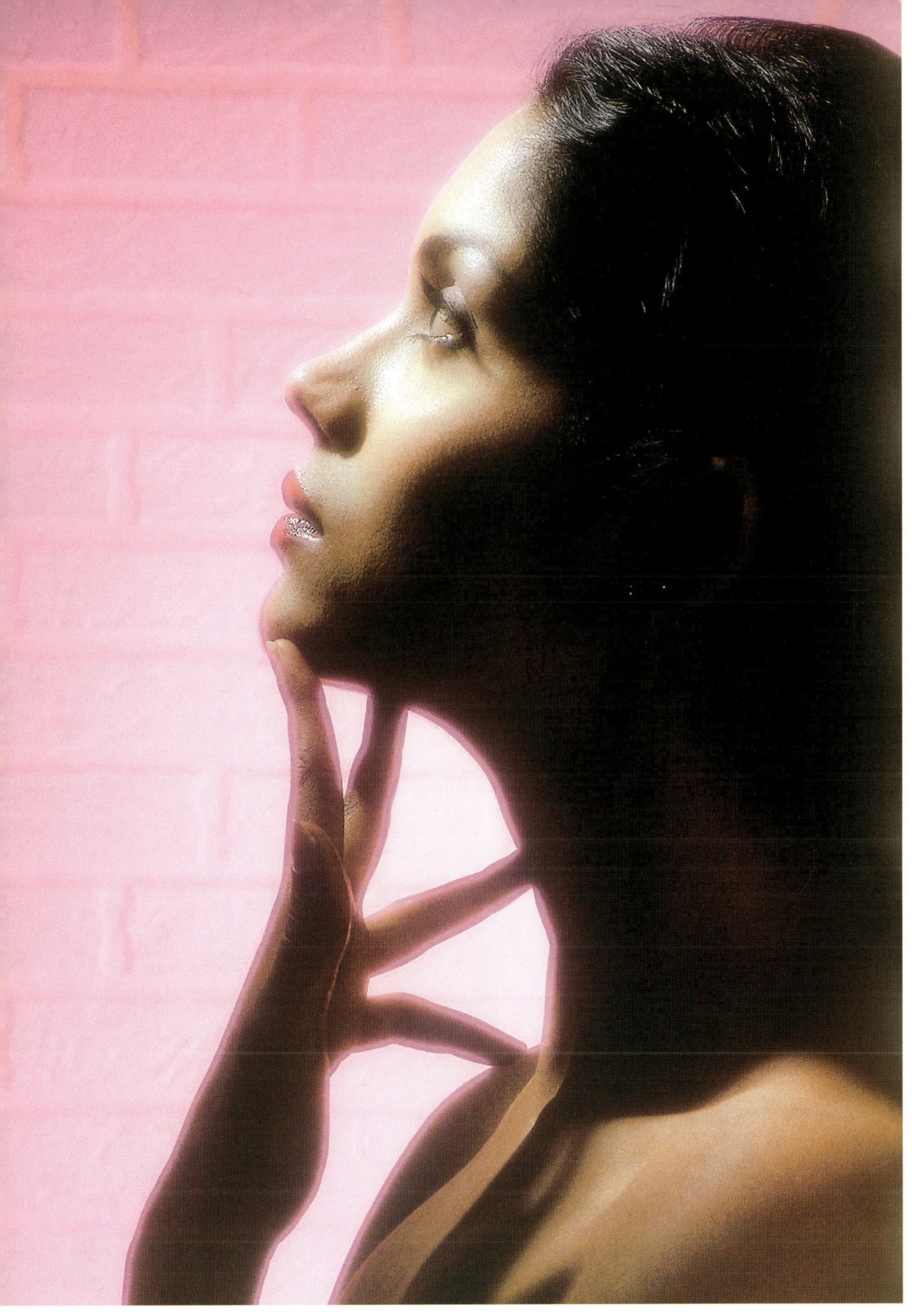

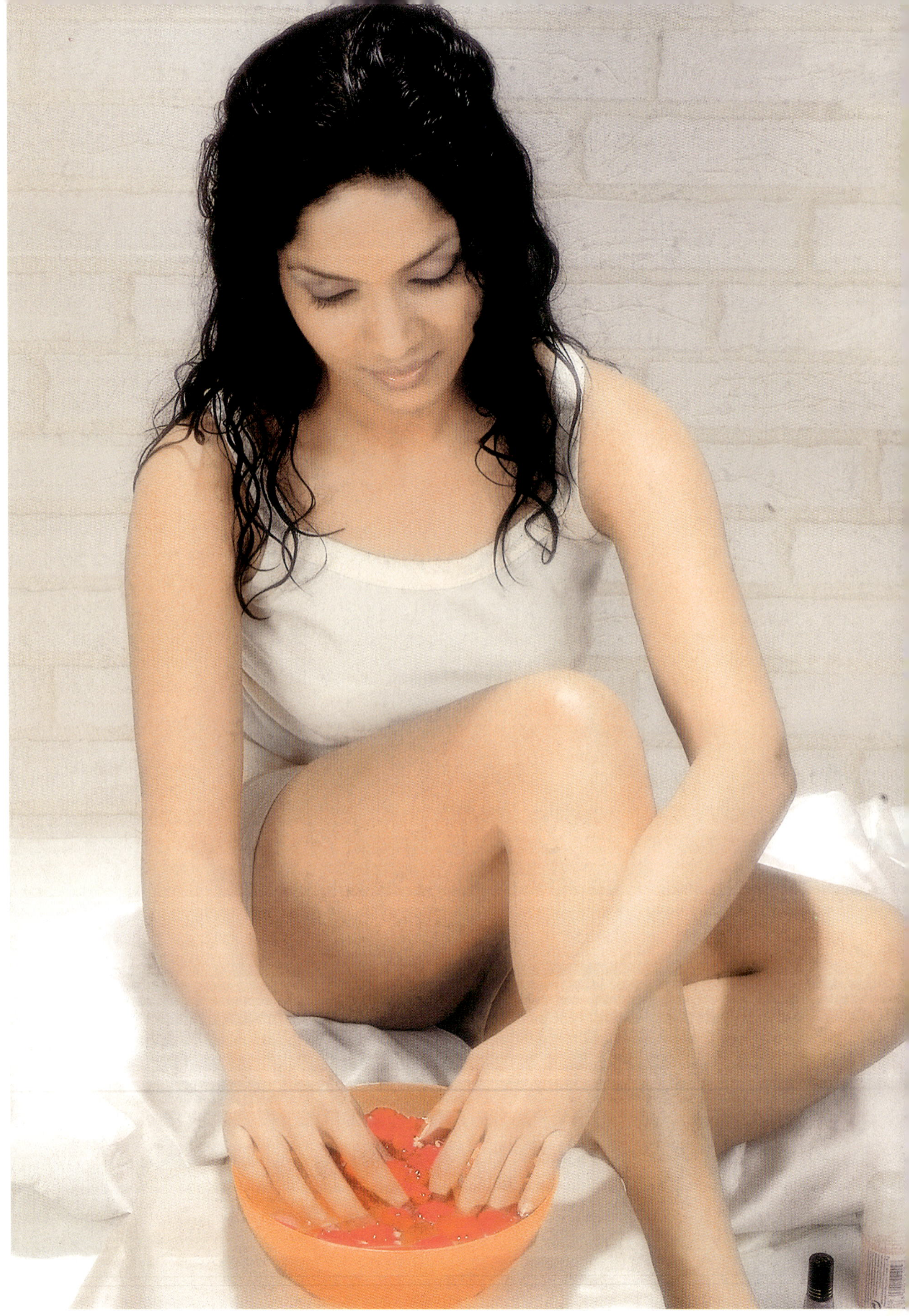

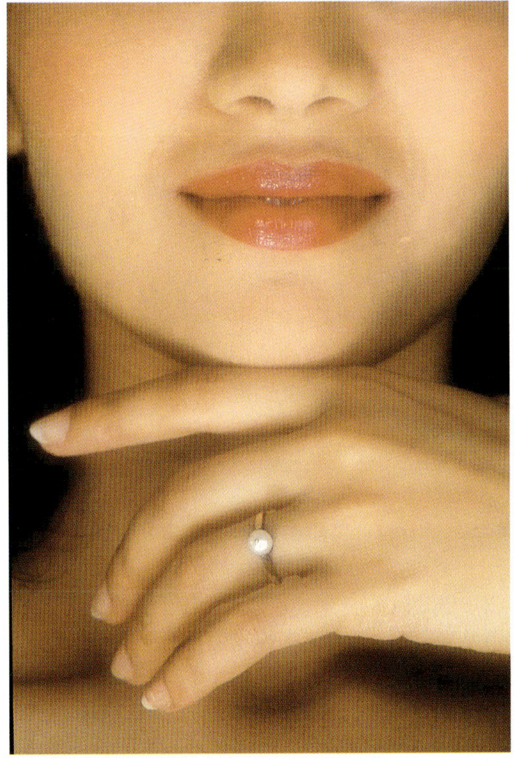

COLD MILK : Did you know that blisters on the hands while cooking can be cured with a cold milk compress if applied immediately? Put some cold milk on the blister; dab it two or three times. It soothes immediately and actually aids in healing.

TURMERIC POWDER : So often hands get minor cuts while chopping vegetables or while performing other household chores. If you havc cut your fingers or hands, immediately apply turmeric powder onto the wound. It stops bleeding and aids healing.

GELATIN : For those people who have split nails and cracked hands, a good 'soak' in gelatin will certainly help. Take a packet of gelatin or lemon jelly, pour it into a cup of hot water. Make a paste and put it to set. When it has set, soak the hands in this jelly, keep rubbing the nails and cuticles as well as the hands. Keep them soaked for at least 15 minutes. A regular use of this treatment prevents cracks on the skin of the fingers and the cracking and splitting of fingernails. Eating jelly also helps promote a healthy growth of nails.

BUTTERMILK AND ALMOND OIL : Take one tablespoon almond oil and one cup buttermilk. Mix well, apply on the hands. Massage well, let it dry, then apply again. Repeat this till all the solution is used up. Use this at night, before bedtime. Wear cotton gloves and sleep. Next morning, rinse well. This treatment ensures that the hands remain soft and maintain a good skin texture.

Nails

Nails require constant care too. They chip, crack and discolour due to harsh treatment. Nails are horny extensions of the skin and are made from the protein called Keratin, like the hair. If the nails are in a poor condition then rough treatment is only a partial cause. Poor or careless nutrition affects the health of nails. Lack of vitamin B and C makes the nails hard and brittle and causes them to crack. An average nail grows by about one millimetre per day. A good diet and sunshine promotes healthy nails.

Nails need to be constantly cleaned, moisturized and buffed to keep them looking healthy. The way you look after your cuticles, the manner in which you file your nails, all these go a long way in promoting a well manicured look. Nails can be irreparably damaged due to cuticle infections, or other damage from housework or use of poor quality soaps and detergents. The cuticles also tend to harden and spread out beyond the nail bed area, further damaging the nails. All these are just due to carelessness and can be overcome by a proper nail care routine.

A nail takes approximately 16 weeks to grow from its root to the tip. Nails cannot miraculously grow overnight, nor can the texture of the hard, yellow, brittle nails change so quickly. A deliberate, patient nail, care routine, combined with the right diet can indeed work wonders and give you perfectly shaped, finely textured nails.

Your nails need to be cleaned gently: Take a sponge soaked in warm water. Squeeze soapy water on your nails and rub on the nails, under the nails, and draw out the dirt. Dry brittle nails should first be soaked in a solution of warm water, olive oil and lime juice. Soak your nails in his solution for 10 minutes, constantly massaging and cleaning your nails, while gently pushing back your cuticles with your fingers. After this cleaning routine, scrub your nails with some good moisturizing cream or lotion. While nail polish does protect the nail and is a good make-over for nails, you should keep your nails free from polish at least once a week, and let them 'breathe' in the air, sunshine and moisture.

Nails need protein to keep them strong. Thus you must take a protein rich diet to prevent them from getting brittle or develop cracks. They should also be kept as dry as possible, and manicured every few days. They should always be kept trimmed to the right length and the cuticles softened and gently pushed back.

Use an emery file (sandpaper) rather than a metal nail file. Do not file away the sides too deeply as one can injure the nail bed.

The colour of your nails is an indicator of good health. Healthy nails are transparent and look a little rosy too. Pale nail beds often indicate anaemia. Yellowing and thickening of nails along with a slow growth rate may be due to illness or lung disease.

Concave nails indicate iron deficiency, while white patches on the nails indicate calcium deficiency. Your diet must be rich and nutritious with plenty of vitamin B as well as calcium, found in whole grains; meat, cottage cheese, green leafy vegetables. Eat garlic daily to keep the nails healthy. A capsule of vitamin E strengthens nails as well.

A few common nail care tips will ensure healthy nails. Keep the nails trimmed, clean and moisture

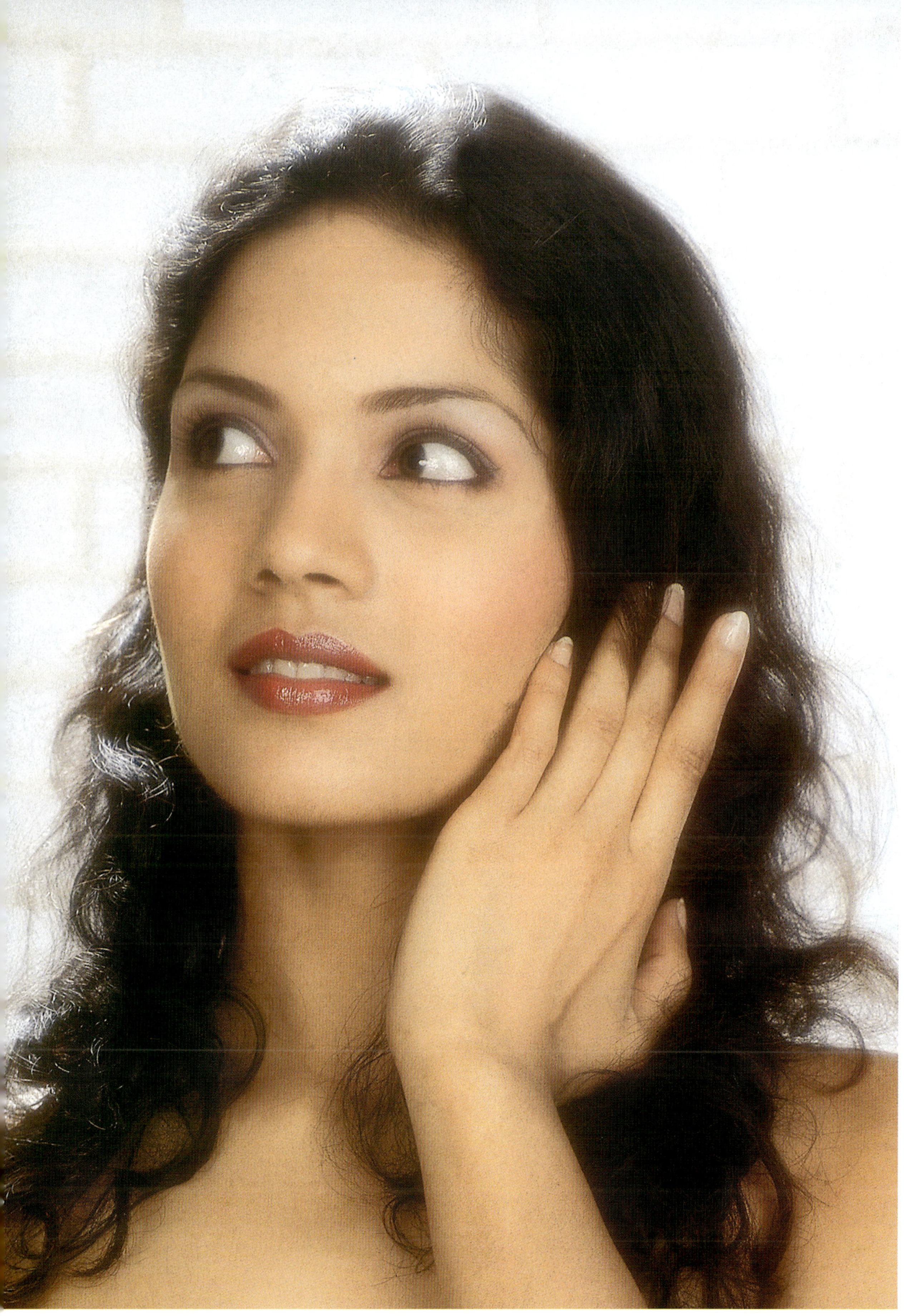

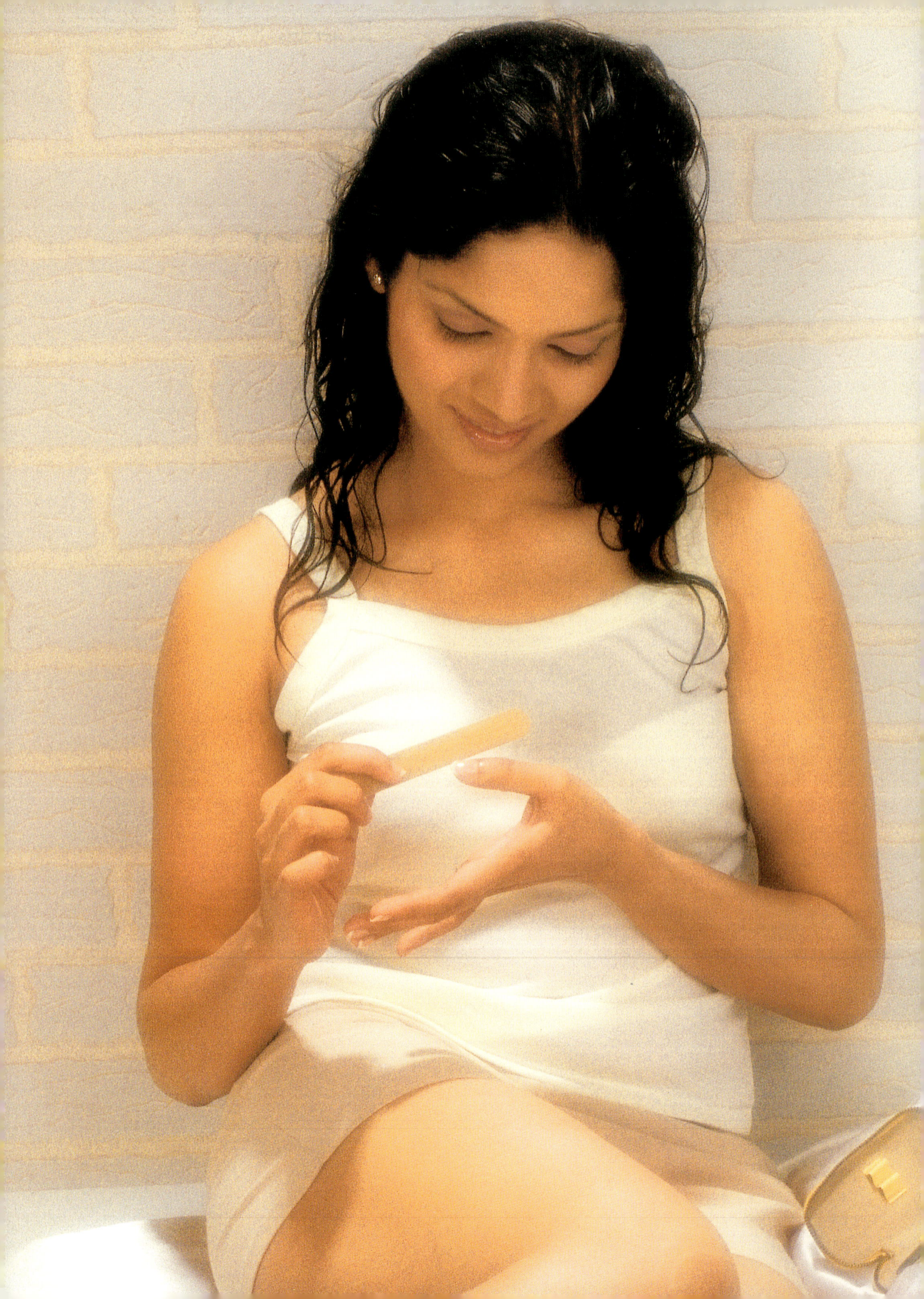

free. Be careful when filing nails, do not file too deeply into the nail bed area to get pointed nails. Use the emery board instead of a metal nail file. Wear gloves while cleaning dishes, swabbing, cleaning or dusting.

Here are some good tips for common nail problems:

TO STRENGTHEN NAILS : Soak daily in warm almond oil or olive oil for 5-7 minutes, preferably before bed-time.

DISCOLOURED NAILS : You can clean discoloured nails by soaking them in a solution of lemon juice and warm water. After 7 minutes, scrub them with white vinegar by using a nail brush.

CRACKED NAILS : To get rid of cracks in nails, apply glycerin at bedtime; rubbing it in generously. Leave it on your hands. It soothes your nails and helps to repair cracks.

SWOLLEN CUTICLES : If your cuticles have swollen and overgrown and are painful, try the following nail care tips:

Soak your hands in warm water for 5 minutes. Make a paste of turmeric powder and sandalwood powder. Apply this paste thickly, like an ointment, on the cuticles. Leave on for 20 minutes and rinse off.

CUTICLE SOFTENER : All you need is one teaspoon warm olive oil or almond oil. After a bath, massage cuticles with warm olive oil or almond oil everyday. While massaging, push back the cuticles, using your fingertip.

TO HARDEN SOFT NAILS : Sometimes soft nails or thin nails crack easily. To harden them, soak them in olive oil for 20 minutes every alternate day.

TO WHITEN NAILS : Dip a swab of cotton wool in hydrogen peroxide; clean the nails with this swab, rub under the nails to clean and whiten them.

The golden rule to a healthy, beautiful pair of hands and lovely nails is protection and care. If you protect your hands and nails and make their care a daily routine, you would see a dramatic improvement. Your hands do not demand expensive creams or lotions, they only demand a little time and attention.

Do not use your nails to open letters! Treat your nails gently, not as 'tools'.

Pamper Your Feet

Women's feet have inspired many poets to pen couplets on them. Popularly called 'lotus feet', a pair of dainty, clean, well shaped feet have indeed been many an owner's pride and a neighbours envy.

There was a time when women were covered from head to toe. In fact, they wore veils and one could not see their faces. The feet were the only visible part of their body. Women's feet have thus inspired many poets to pen couplets on them. Popularly called 'lotus feet' a pair of dainty, clean, well shaped feet have indeed been many an owner's pride.

To own a pair of soft, lovable, beautiful feet you need to pamper them by creaming and massaging them regularly. Dry rough nails, fungal infection, cracked heels, swollen feet, corns, calluses are all the result of years of neglect. How thoughtlessly we ensnare them in a pair of ill-fitting sandals or shoes that only seem to pinch, hurt and maul. This ends up disfiguring your feet, causing back problems and poor posture apart from disrupting blood ciruclation.

By following a few careful do's and don'ts you can look after your feet. First, some basic rules:

Bathing, massaging and exercising your feet, and giving them a pedicure are the very basic necessities that go a long way in ensuring that your feet remain soft, shapely and supple.

The first golden rule is to buy shoes of the right size. Apart from the size, you have to ensure that the length of heels that you are buying, does not destabilize you. People with bad backs should not wear pencil heels that hurt the spine. One should buy shoes in the afternoon or evening when the feet are swollen from the day's walking. This will ensure that you get the right fit and size.

Next is exercising your feet. Most people believe that just because they are 'on their feet' the whole day, they have exercised their feet. This is far from true. You need to exercise to relax your tired feet and to strengthen your foot muscles. The best time to exercise is at the end of the day.

Sit comfortably on an erect chair and clench your toes, then relax them—do this four to six times a day. Then stretch your toes and ankles, pull them back and release them.

Next draw circles in the air with your feet. Move one foot at a time, first clockwise, then anti-clockwise five to six times. This exercises your ankles, keeping them supple and lean.

Besides exercise, you should specially bathe your feet daily. Normally when one has a bath, the body, face and arms get all the attention—the feet remain neglected. So, make it a habit of treating your feet to a lavish footbath, especially at the end of the day.

Take a basin of warm water to which a little salt has been added. Soak your feet in this. Your aching feet will get instant relief. Pat dry your feet thoroughly. Apply a lotion of glycerin and rosewater and dry your feet and apply talc later. Once a week indulge yourself in a good pedicure. You can easily do this at home.

Every day, after you have cleaned and exercised your feet, put them 'up' (literally). Take a round bolster. Lie down flat without a pillow. Now place your ankles on the edge of the bolster so as to raise your feet. Keep in this position for at least 15 minutes. This gives immediate relief to tired feet. Its also

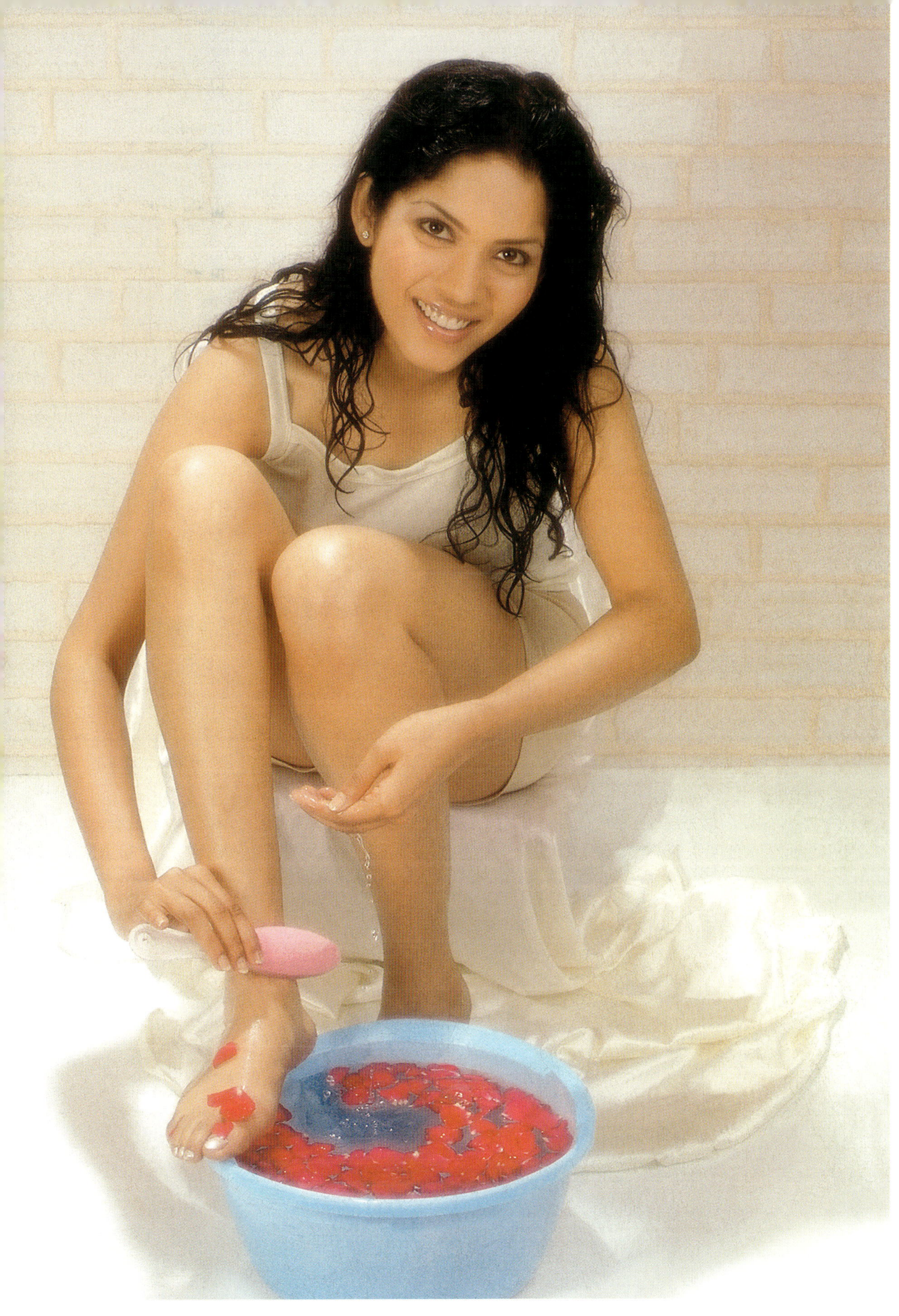

helps reduce swelling due to water retention. Last, but not least, while bathing, remove dead skin with a pumice stone and loofah.

Our feet keep us balanced and carry our weight. In a lifetime they walk as much as going five times around the earth. We only pay attention to our feet when they rebel at their utter neglect; when they can bear the neglect no longer and become ill with calluses, corns, bruises and ingrown toenails and bunions. We should look after our feet before any of these problems creep in. Some of the serious foot problems may need the attention of a doctor. So, prevention is always better than cure. You can certainly prevent a lot of foot problems by knowing about them and preventing them by using the right home cures. So take a look at your feet and start caring for them right away.

Now let us discuss a few common foot problems and how we can tackle them.

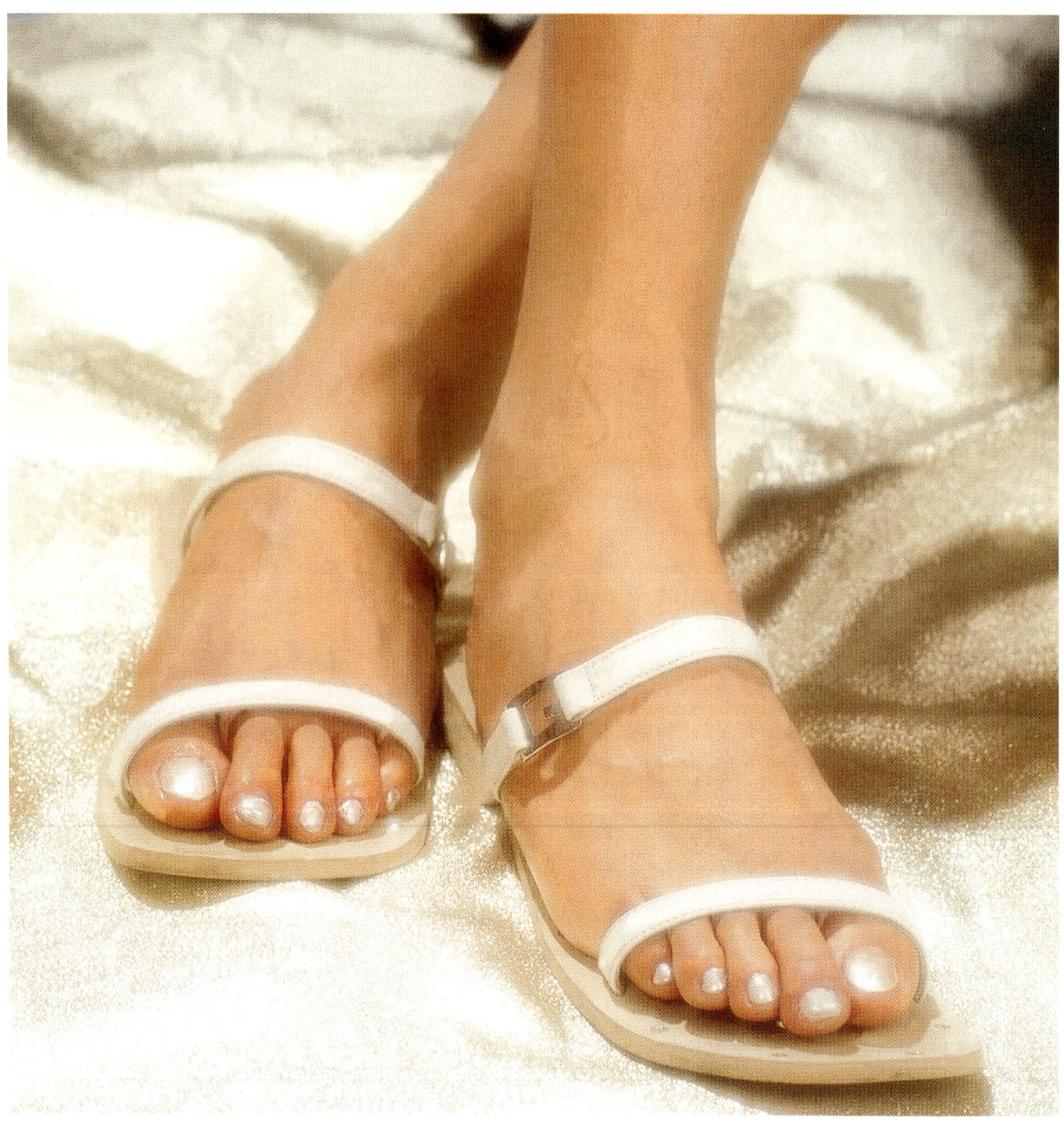

Neglected Feet

Most foot problems arise due to neglect and oversight. Cracked feet, corns and other common ailments should be attended to and nipped in the bud. A few suggestions to deal with them.

Cracked Heels

This is one of the most common and embarrassing problems. Cracked heels are the first signs of sheer neglect. A daily dose of cleansing and moisturizing will help.

Before going to bed, soak your feet in warm soapy water for 15 minutes. Wash and dry. Then take one teaspoon Vaseline. Add to it the juice of one lemon. Rub this mixture into the cracked heels and other areas of the feet till it is thoroughly absorbed. This should be done daily.

A mixture of glycerin and rosewater too, if applied regularly, helps to soothe and cure cracked-heels.

FOOT EXFOLIANTS AND SCRUBS

You need to exfoliate your feet without being too harsh. Dead skin accumulated on the feet can cause a lot of problems. The ideal way to get rid of calluses is to exfoliate. Use a loofah at least twice a day to get rid of the dead skin. However, nourishing and exfoliating your feet should be done every week.

STRAWBERRY EXFOLIATES : Take 6-8 strawberries and two tablespoons of olive (or almond) oil, and one teaspoon of sea-salt.

Mash the strawberries. Add the oil and salt. Make into a paste. Massage into the feet, rubbing harshly as you go along. Keep rubbing, especially around the hardened areas of your feet. Leave the paste on for 10-15 minutes. Rinse with warm water, then with cold water.

Another good exfoliate is to use crushed almonds, instead of strawberries. Both exfoliate the tough skin of your feet and the natural juices and oils nourish your feet.

Other natural exfoliating foot scrubs can be prepared by grinding corncobs and walnut shells. These are especially good for exfoliating very toughened feet, especially the heel areas.

ORANGE AND OIL SCRUB : This is an ideal cooling foot scrub. Take two oranges, one cup of oil (any vegetable oil will do), and one cup of sea salt.

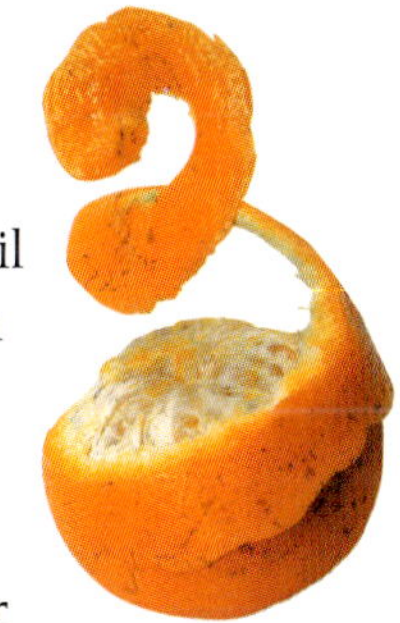

Mix together salt and oil. Thickly slice the oranges into rings. Dip them into this oil and salt lotion and start rubbing all over the feet. Use generously on the hardened skin areas. Keep rubbing vigorously for 10 minutes, then rinse off. This cleans your feet, cools and softens them.

Calluses on the feet can also be cured by rubbing the soles of the feet with lemon sliced into half. Take a lemon, slice it into half, and rub it vigorously in circular motions over the toes, heels and other tough and hard areas.

Corns

These are caused by friction and pressure when the bony parts of your feet rub against your shoes. The problem needs to be treated by a doctor. Change your footwear immediately. Use exfoliates, warm footbaths and moisturizing routines to ease the pain. There are a few home cures too that can cure newly formed corns. They should be treated at once. Any delay will require the attention of doctor.

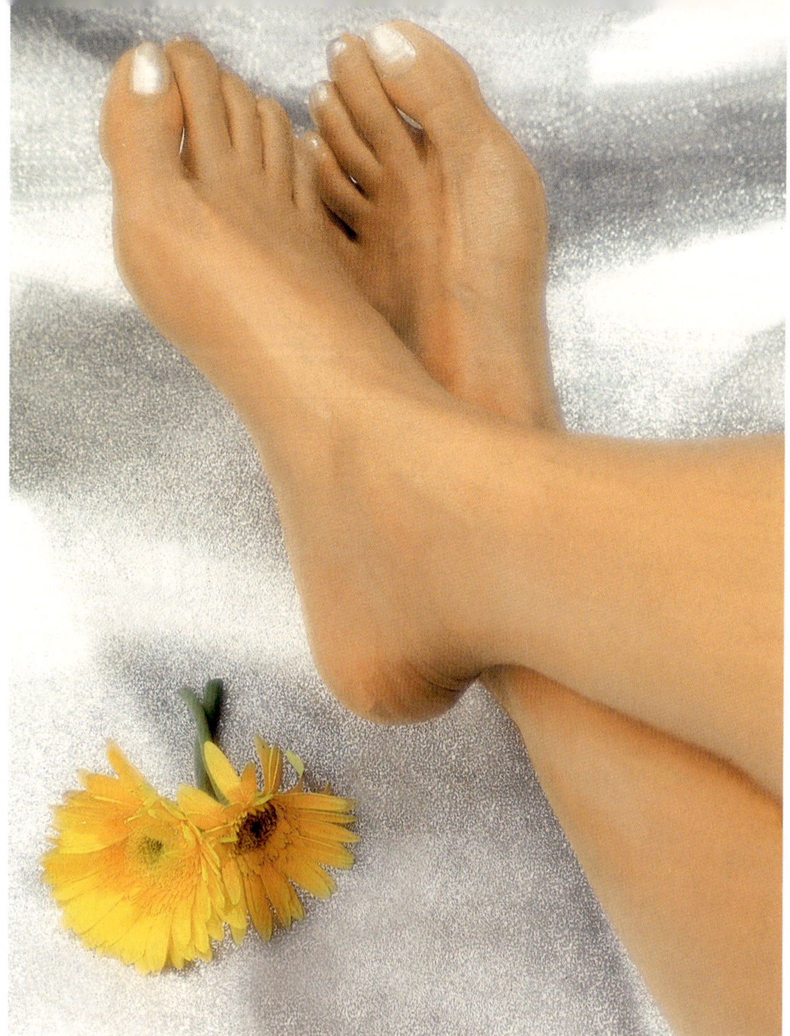

MARIGOLD : The marigold flower belongs to the same family as the arnica. It has antiseptic qualities. The juice of the leaves is an excellent cure for warts. The sap from its stem is useful in curing warts, corns and calluses of the feet.

All one has to do is to slice the stem lengthwise and apply the juice of the stem on the affected areas. Leave it on. Use this treatment everyday at the first sight of the corn.

LICORICE : The dried roots of this plant and its underground stems are used as flavouring agents in food as well as the base in many cough medicines.

Take a few licorice sticks; powder them and add a little mustard oil. Rub this paste onto the corns and the hardened skin. Use regularly, especially at bedtime. Leave it on. All newly formed corns will disappear.

PINEAPPLE : This is an absolutely unique way to treat corns. At night, just before bedtime, soak your feet in warm water for 20 minutes to tenderize the corns. Cut out a square piece from the pineapple peel. Rest the inside of this directly on the corn. Use tape to attach this piece directly on the corn. Cover with socks and leave on overnight. Apply for four or five nights consecutively. This would be of great help in treating the corn. Pineapple contains an enzyme called Brometain that softens and breaks down dead skin. So don't throw away that pineapple peel. Use it to cure painful corns.

Swollen Feet

Sometimes, mild water retention or odema, especially during the menstrual cycle or due to hormonal changes can cause immense discomfort. Here is a simple cure.

CARROT AND PARSLEY JUICE : Take four carrots, one beetroot or apple, and a few sprigs of parsley. Wash, peel and finely chop the carrots and also the apple or beetroot. Add a few sprigs of parsley. Blend in a juicer, strain. Drink this juice twice a day to treat bloated feet.

Athletes Foot

This is one of the most common and irritating foot infections. This usually spreads through wet socks, bedding or bathrooms of swimming pools. This infection spreads due to dampness. The best thing to do is to keep your feet dry. Here is a useful home remedy:

GINGER OR GARLIC : Soak your feet in a basin of warm water containing either a few pods of crushed garlic or crushed ginger. Add to this a little alcohol. Soak feet for 10 minutes. Remove feet and dry them thoroughly. Repeat 2-3 times a day. This provides immense relief.

An all-purpose foot cream can easily be prepared at home too.

COCO-ROSE FOOT CREAM : Take half cup coconut oil, one teaspoon glycerin and two tablespoons rose water. Take a mixing bowl and pour all these ingredients together. Beat till a smooth paste is formed. Store in a jar and keep it in your bathroom. Use every night to prevent drying of the feet and cracks in the feet. Its an ideal, multi-purpose foot care cream.

Shoe Bites

We often suffer from shoe bites. These can occur due to wearing new or ill-fitting shoes. Whenever you buy a new pair of shoes, use these preventive measures to prevent shoe bites.

Apply a little petroleum jelly inside your shoe. Leave it on overnight. Clean it off with a cloth and then wear your shoes.

Apply coconut oil inside your shoes for three consecutive nights to soften them before wearing. You could apply castor oil too.

Apply some raw potato slices inside the shoe and particularly the heel area. Repeat for two nights before wearing your new shoes:

In case you still get a shoe bite, try the following:

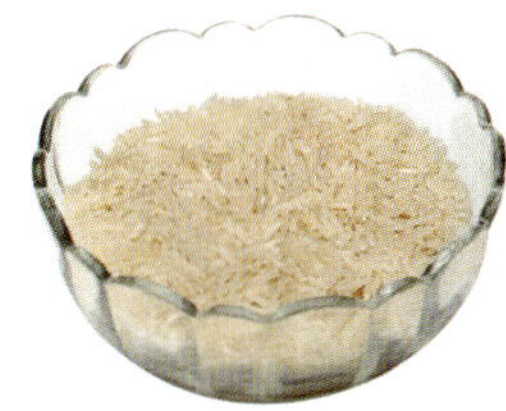

RICE : Take half cup rice. Pound it to a powder and then add enough water to make a thick paste. Apply the paste on the shoe bite. Leave it on till dry. Rinse gently with lukewarm water. Dry the feet thoroughly. You will get immense relief.

NEEM AND TURMERIC PASTE : Take a few neem leaves and add to them a tablespoon of turmeric powder. Add a little water and put it into mixer to form a thick paste. Apply this paste on the painful shoe bite. This gives tremendous relief and also dries up the bite.

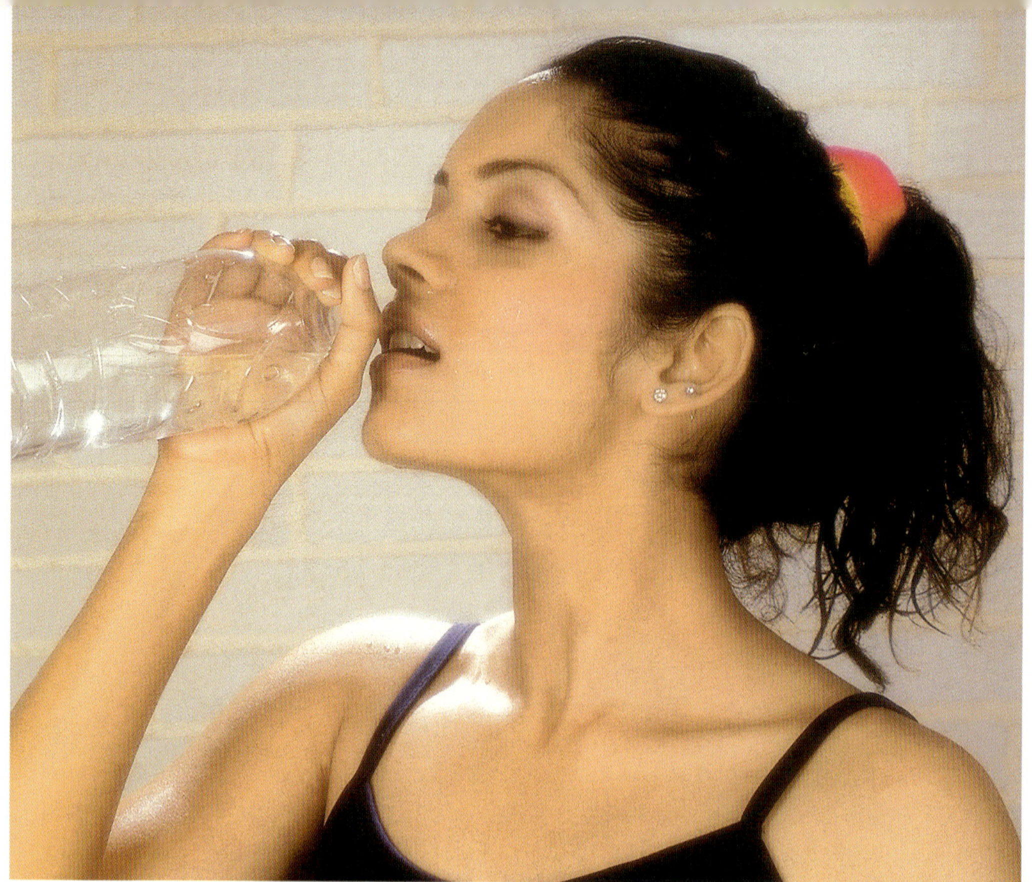

Helpful Tips

Potions, conditioners and nourishers need to be replenished with a few healthy habits. These tips will enhance the beauty and health of your skin.

* Drink at least 2 litres of water everyday to flush out toxins.
* Start your day by having a glass of warm water to which you add a few drops of honey and lemon juice. This cleans and purifies your blood and imparts a glow to your skin.
* During the course of your day, clean your skin as often as possible. Just frequent splashes of water and a brisk rub of the towel are enough to generate circulation.
* Don't overload the skin with heavy make-up.
* To reduce body hair, use this quick and easy formula. Take half cup chickpea powder. Add 1 teaspoon of turmeric powder and 1 tablespoon of any oil. Make a thick paste. Apply all over arms, legs, etc. Let it dry. Use circular motion to remove the paste. If you use this paste regularly, your bodily hair will thin down considerably.
* Soak in the early rays of the sun. It is very good for your health and rejuvenation.
* Pollution robs your skin of its natural moisture. Thus to combat this effect, on reaching home wash your hands and face and exposed parts of the body with cold water. Immediately rub cold milk, or glycerin and rose water on these parts to soothe them.
* Once in month go for a professional massage.
* Don't let your hands and feet pay the price for your lack of time. Both are very visible parts of your body. A few minutes devoted to their care would give amazing results.

  Remember, to manicure and pedicure them every week.

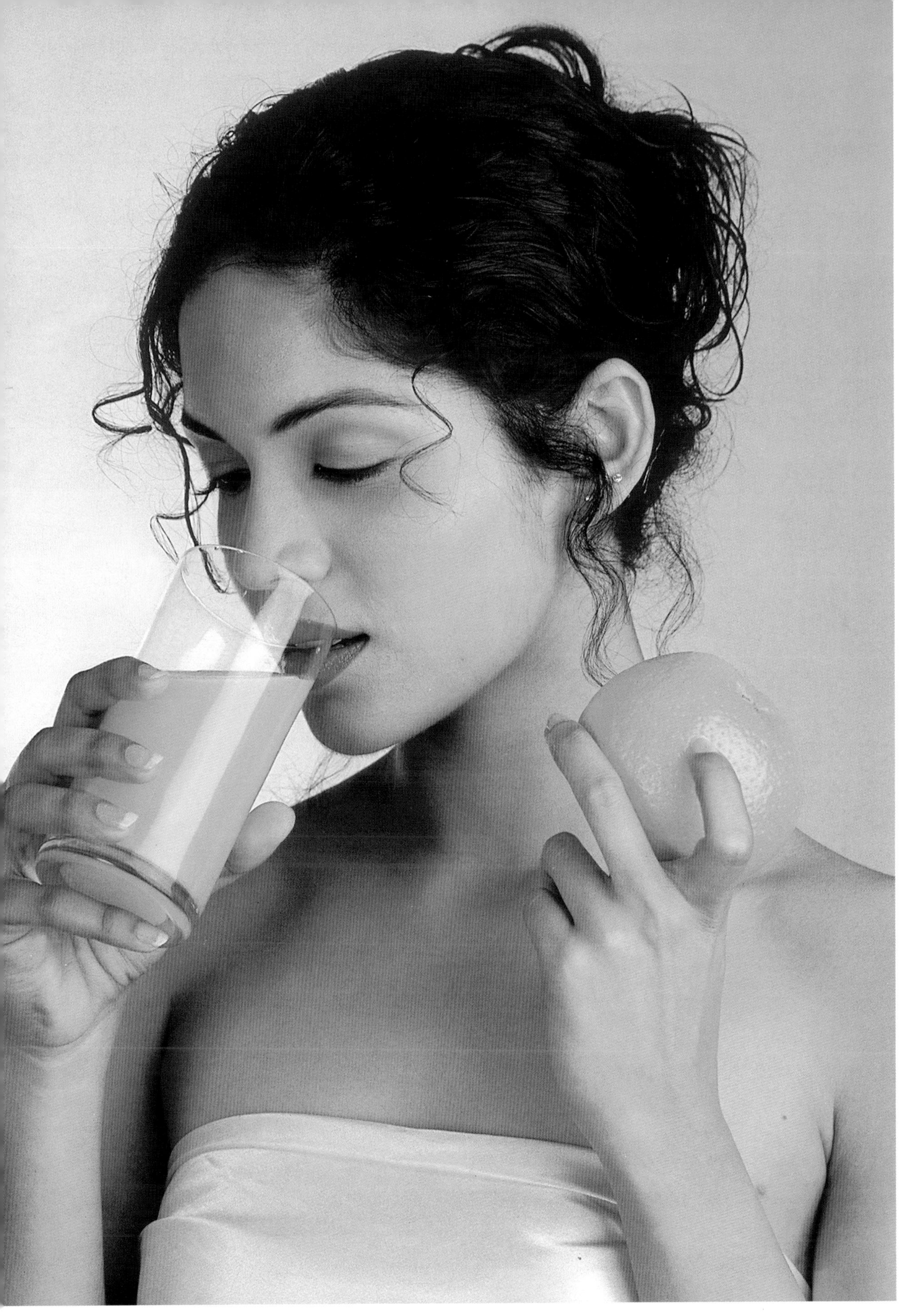

* MANICURE

At home you need:

- A bowl of mild soapy water
- Nail clippers
- Emery board
- Cotton wool
- Nail buffer or a baby toothbrush
- Vaseline to soften the cuticles
- Orange stick with tip wrapped in cotton wool

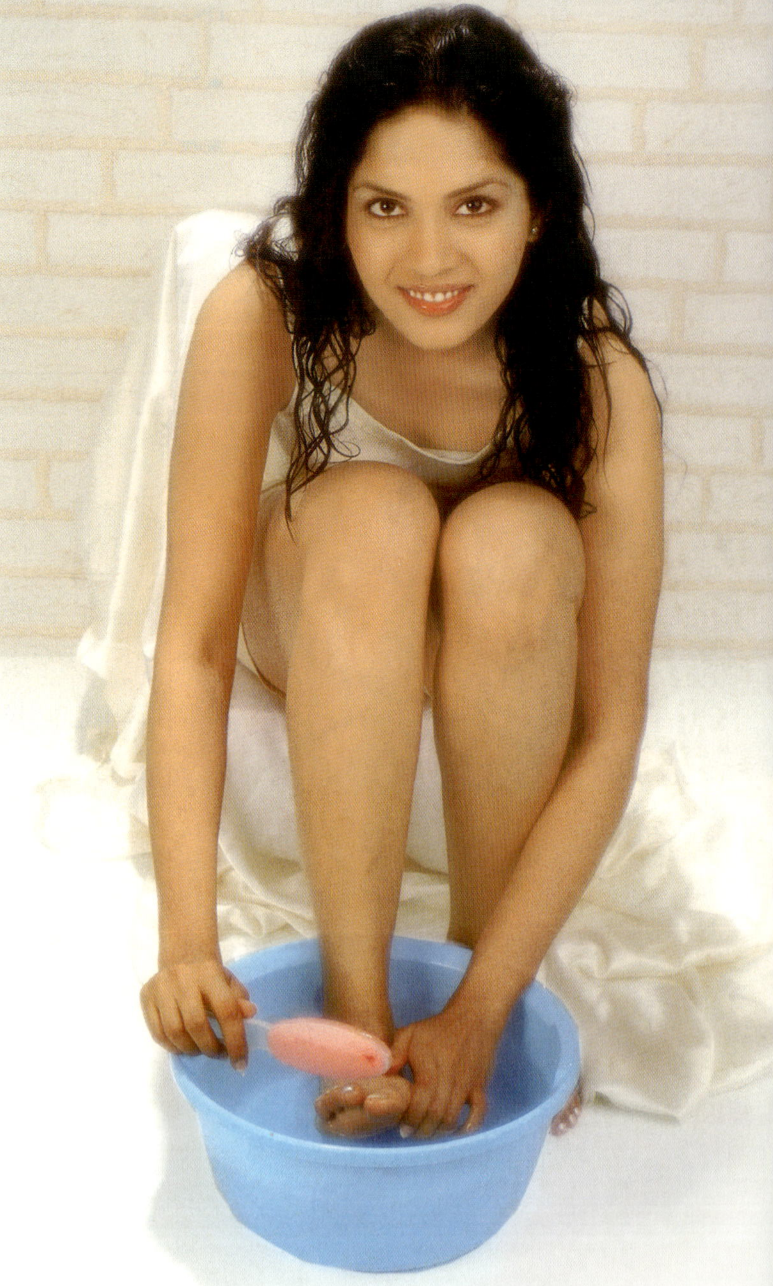

First clip your nails if required. Use the emery boards to file your nails into a smooth oval shape. Use single stroke for filing.

Remove nail polish with a nail polish remover.

Rinse your hands in water. Use the toothbrush and the soapy water to gently scrub the nails clean. Rinse your hands in cold water and pat dry.

Apply nail polish if desired.

Nail polish should be applied in 3 strokes. The first stroke should be up the centre from the cuticle to the nail tip, the second and third on either sides.

Do not overlook any pain, swelling, itching or redness in your hands and feet. Identify the cause and treat it immediately.

While filing your nails do not use a see-saw motion. File them lightly with feather strokes in one direction only.

If your nails are brittle, then eat lots of jelly.

Sterilize your manicure and pedicure equipment with alcohol after each use.

A few additional tips:

- Exercise fingers by curling them tightly and opening them.
- Knitting helps to exercise your fingers.
- Use a pumice stone and loofah everyday at bath time to get rid of calluses and any rough spots on the feet.
- The best time to push back cuticles is at bath time when they are soaked in water and have softened.
- Don't throw away lemon peels; rub them on your toenails and finger nails. They are natural cleansers.

* PEDICURE

At home you need:

- A small tub of warm, soapy water to soak your feet
- Pumice stone
- Baby toothbrush
- Rosewater and glycerin lotion
- Nail clippers
- Emery board
- Orange stick
- Nail polish remover
- Nail polish
- Talcum powder

Soak your feet in the warm, soapy water for about 10 minutes. Remove any dirt under the toe nails with a soft toothbrush. Remove from water and dry your feet well with a soft towel.

Use the pumice stone to remove thick, dry or dead skin from your heels or the sides of your feet.

Soak feet again for 5 minutes and then dry them.

- Massage feet with generous amount of moisturizer.
- Clip and file toenails.
- Remove nail polish if any.
- Push back the cuticle with orange stick whose tips are wrapped in cotton wool.
- Apply nail polish if desired.

face
Reflects Your Aura

Oriental women as well as those from Egypt, Rome and other ancient civilizations were known for their tremendous skills in beauty care. As the Italian writer Sonnini says about oriental women, in his book *Travels*: "Nowhere are the women more beautiful, nowhere are they better skilled or more practiced in the art of arresting or repairing the ravages of time." Indeed, oriental women have always exuded an aura of beauty. The aura of your personality is directly reflected on your face. It is one of the most expressive and delicate parts of your body — it also bears the onslaught of age and weather more than any other part of the body. It therefore needs to be preserved and protected most preciously.

A beautiful face can be described as one which is cared for and which awakens admiration for that reason. From the earliest civilizations, women have searched for and used beauty cures and aids. Today, perfectly generated beauty cures are available and beauty culture is an enormous business, as can be seen from vast advertising budgets. Launches of beauty products are done on a very lavish scale. All kinds of incentives are offered to lure women to a product. Whenever women flip through a magazine, watch films or ramp shows, they wish that they too had the perfectly sculpted body and flawless skin like the models they see. Few women however realise that what they see is a perfectly "made-up" face and not necessarily a flawless beauty. Care for your skin can enable you to look beautiful. To make your face have the ability to "launch a thousand ships" and to acquire a beautiful and blemish-free skin, you need to pamper it.

"Back to nature" is the global mantra of beauty care today. You can enhance your beauty with the help of products provided by nature itself.

In ancient times too beauty care stemmed from nature. Perfumes made from flowers, barks of scented wood were mixed with oils and left to mature. Once the oils and the wood absorbed the fragrance of these flowers, they were converted to perfumes and scented oils for the body and face. These were lavishly used to prevent the skin from drying, and to protect it from the harsh elements of nature.

Women and men too, extensively used make-up in ancient times. Eye paint made from green

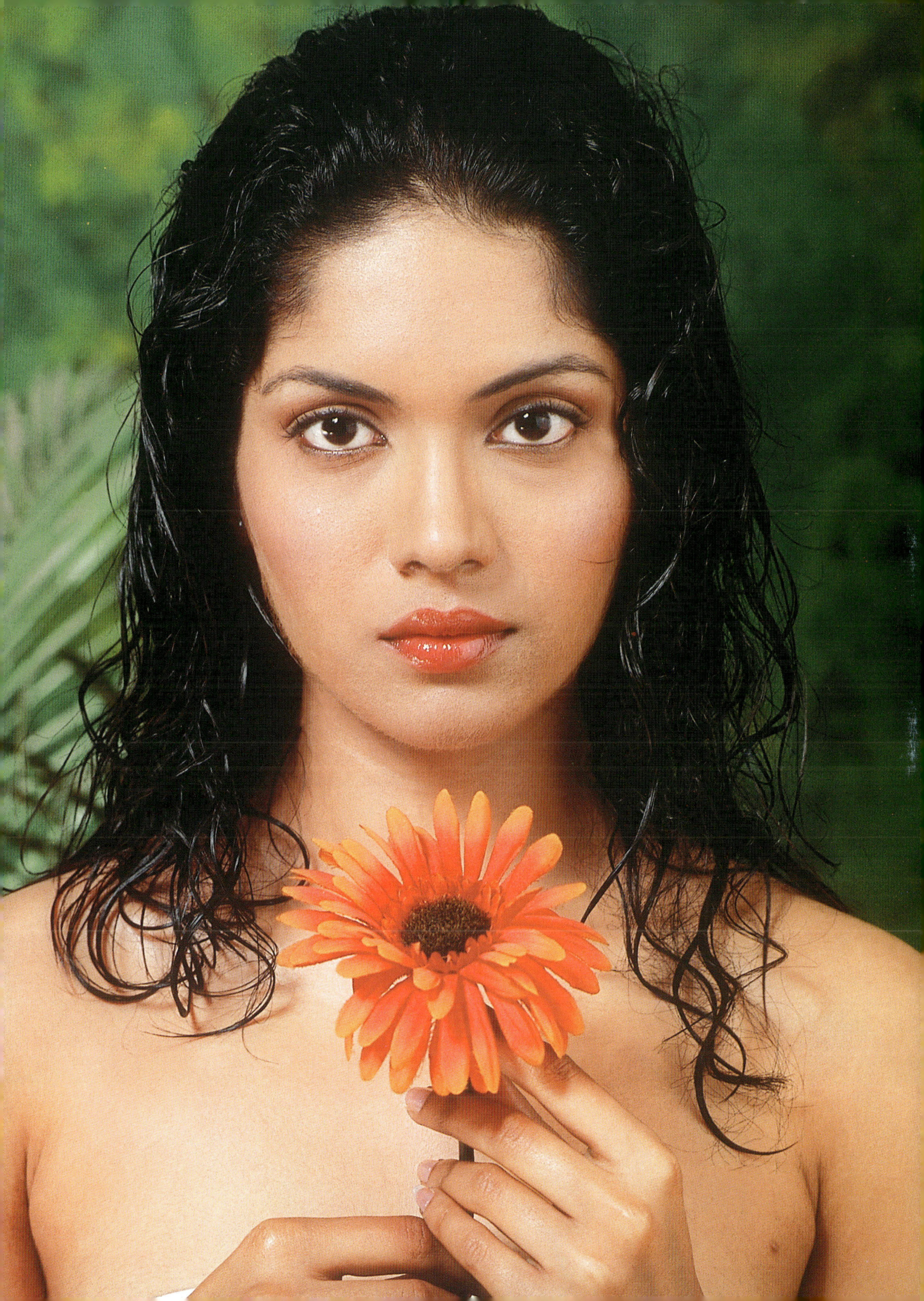

malachite, grey ore, and galena was ground to a powder and mixed with oil to form kohl for the eyes.

Colour for lips, cheeks and nails was made from red ochre clay. Powders for whitening the face were used by Assyrian women even as long back as in 1000 BC. Special make-up jars, beautifully carved bottles made from stone and glass were used to store cosmetics. Thus, women in ancient times managed to look stunning without using any chemical-based or synthetic cosmetics which did not exist then.

Over the years, man developed mass-produced, synthetic beauty products. Contrary to their purpose, these have sometimes caused more problems than what they set out to cure. In fact, many doctors and cosmetologists believe that a number of skin problems can be attributed to synthetic beauty products. As a result, people are again moving towards natural beauty aids. Eco-friendly, natural cosmetics and beauty products are now in great demand. These truly enhance the quality of your skin and so make you look and feel healthier and lovelier.

Nature's bounty has provided us with a treasure chest, which if used effectively can bring out that special glow in your face. It is not necessary to spend a fortune to look beautiful. You can work wonders by just delving into your home's treasure trove of fruits, flowers,vegetables and condiments to find the right cure.

You must also accept yourself and turn your so-called "flaws" into features of your personality. For instance, a sharp pointed nose, or freckles or a mole on your cheek need not be camouflaged; any or all of these can become a distinctive part of your personality, to be used as an advantage. Besides, most common problems can be cured at home. Do you have under-eye shadows? Are you worried about wrinkles? What about pimples? Head towards the kitchen and help yourself to its bounty, which if used the right way could well be that Alladin's lamp which lights up your beautiful face.

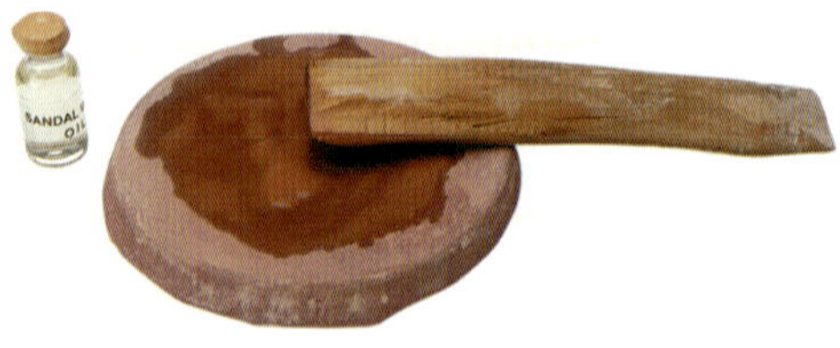

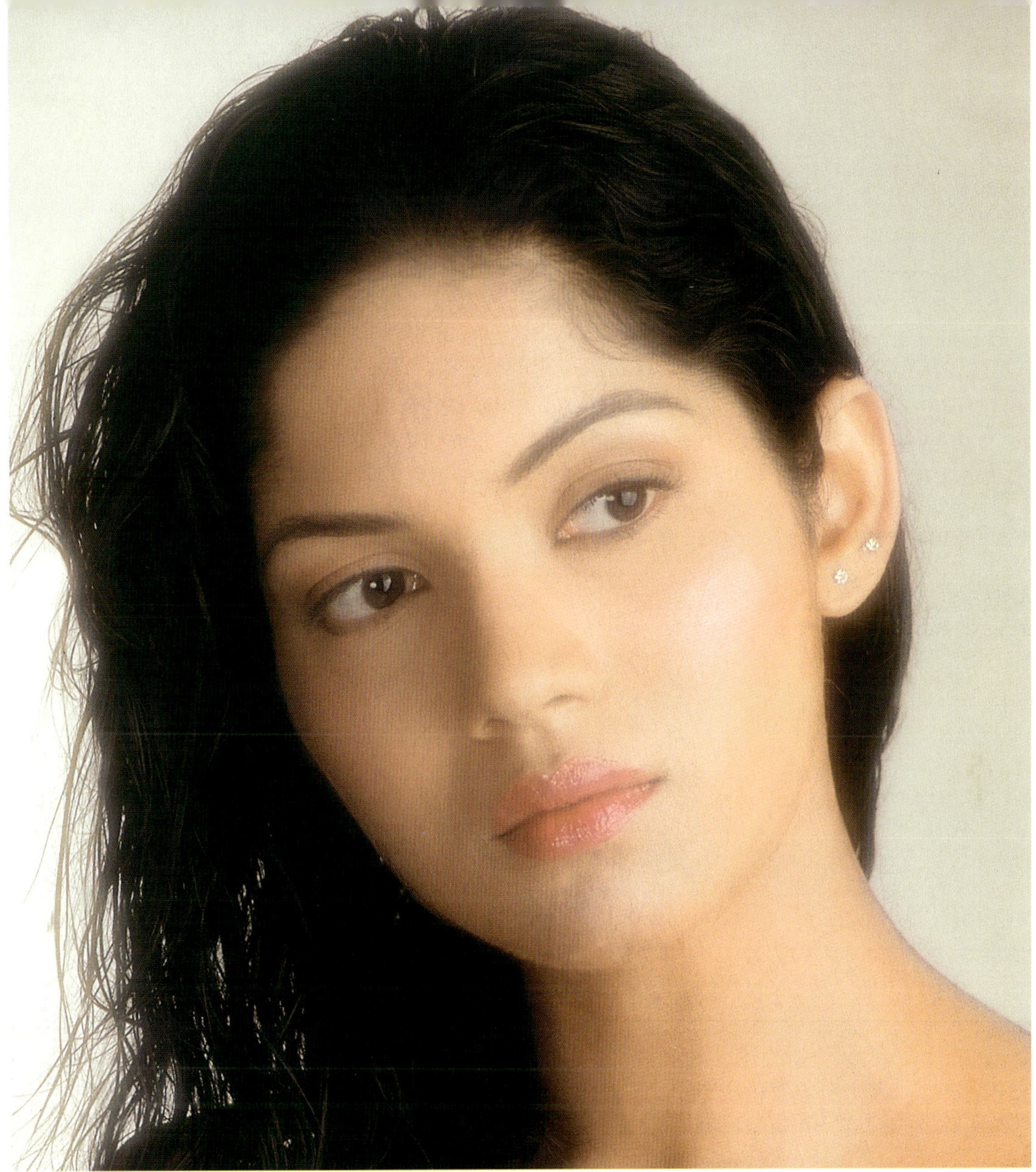

Skin Problems

Facial Facts

Some of the most common problems that women have are related to the skin. Freckles, dry skin, wrinkles, pimples and oily skin, shadows — the list is endless. A little knowledge of their causes and prevention can go a long way in combating them. Some problems are genetic while others are merely a part of the ageing process. Today, women face a host of hair and skin problems. This is mainly due to poor food habits, a disorganised lifestyle and of course, environmental pollution. Here we would like to deal with some of these problems and suggest some really wonderful home cures for them.

Today, international beauty houses are being compelled to use natural products as the modern, health and beauty conscious woman is going back to nature. These cures yield better and longer lasting results. They enhance the beauty of your face and radiate that special aura from within you.

Cleansers

Face care begins with a good wash. Cleansing creams and lotions are used to remove stale make-up and dirt. If this is not regularly done, then the pores get clogged leading to numerous skin problems. Here are some easy to make, and even easier to use, face cleansers suitable for different types of skin.

CHICKPEA POWDER AND TURMERIC : Take half cup chickpea powder. Add one teaspoon turmeric powder and half cup of milk. Stir well. Apply this paste all over the forehead, face and neck. Wait for two minutes and wash off. This is good for oily or mixed skin types. The chickpea powder absorbs the extra oil and the milk nourishes your skin, leaving it tingling fresh.

MILK : Nature's most effective natural cleanser. Take half a cup of cold milk. Add half teaspoon of salt. Stir. Take balls of cotton, soak and then gently dab milk and salt lotion all over forehead, face, and

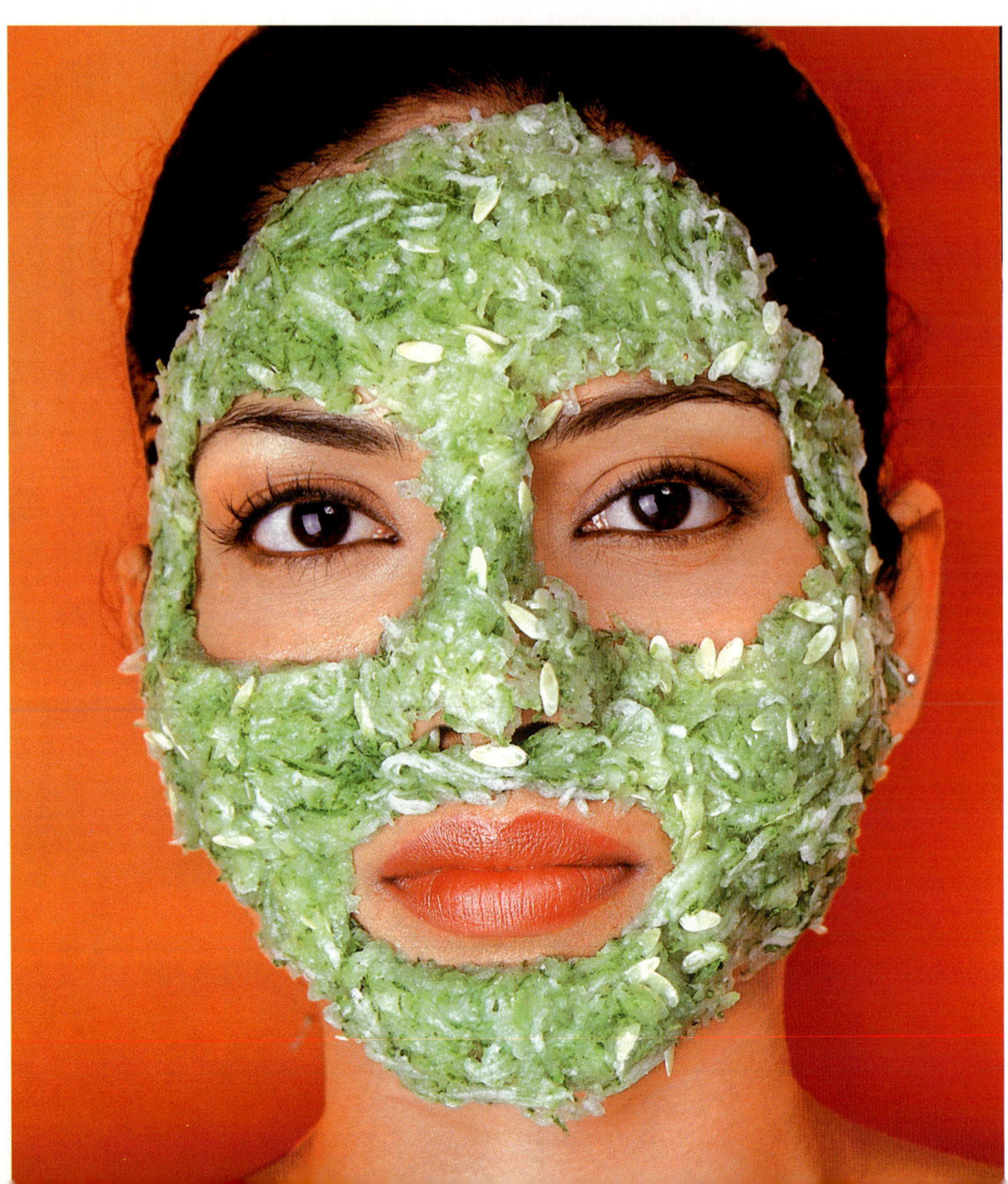

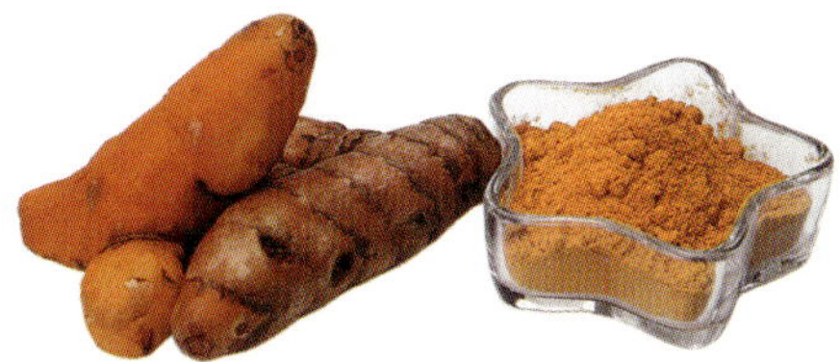

neck. Leave it on for 2–3 minutes. Apply again. Now rub gently in circular motions and wash off. The salt in the milk gently exfoliates dead skin and the milk nourishes the skin. Your face instantly gets a fresh and glowing look. This is good for all skin types.

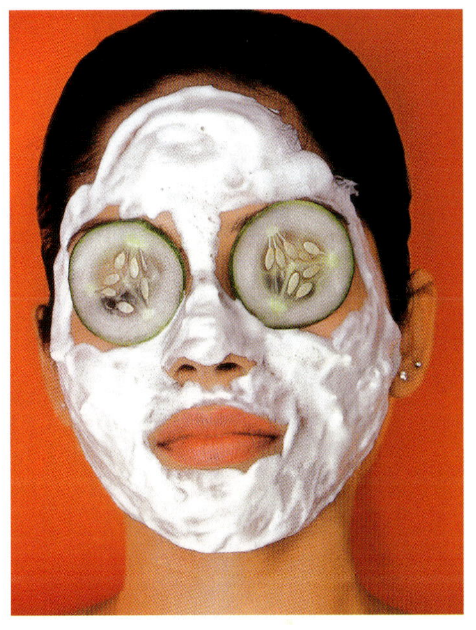

CUCUMBER AND CURD : Take one cucumber, grate it. Squeeze out the juice. Add to this 3–4 tablespoons of beaten curds. Stir well. Apply this paste all over the forehead, face and neck. Leave it on for 3–4 minutes. Wash face and neck with cold water. While cleaning and tightening the pores, it also lightens blemishes and freckles. Very nourishing for the skin. You could use just grated cucumber as a face cleanser too.

YOGHURT : This is yet another effective face cleanser, very good for dry skin. Take half a cup yoghurt. Add to this half teaspoon honey. Stir well. Apply all over the forehead, face and neck. Rub it in gently. Leave on for 2–3 minutes. Wash off with cold water.

CHAMOMILE : Take a handful of fresh chamomile flowers. Add to these some rosemary tops, fresh or dry. Boil them well in a pan containing 2 cups of water. Let the mixture cool. Mash flowers well. Strain and keep. When cool, dip in small pieces of muslin, wring and apply all over the forehead, face and neck. Keep dipping and applying several times. Let it dry. Wash off when completely dry. An excellent cleanser.

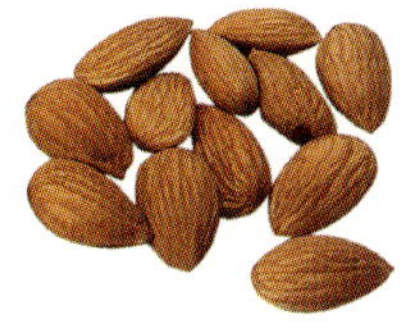

ALMOND : Take 5–7 almonds. Pound them to a paste/powder. Take the yolk of one egg. Beat it up. Add to it one tablespoon of honey and continue beating. Now add almond paste/powder. Mix well. Apply all over the forehead, face and neck. Rub it in gently. When it begins to dry, wash off with lukewarm water. Good for dry skins, especially in winter when the skin tends to lose its natural oils. This acts as a restorative.

HONEY AND VITAMIN A/E : This is a very good and effective cleanser, especially for people with blemishes. Take half cup warm water. Add one-tablespoon honey. Snip open one capsule of vitamin A and one capsule of vitamin E. Mix well. Apply quickly all over the face. Leave it on for 2 minutes and wash with cold water.

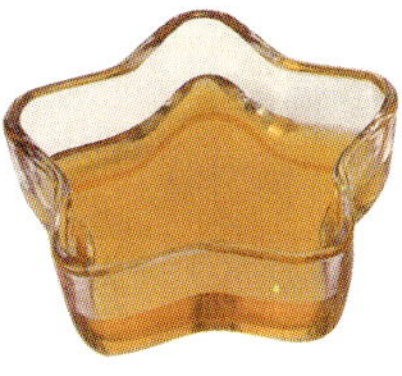

These cleansers can be used in the mornings before a bath, however, it is imperative to use them at bedtime. Remove all traces of make-up with milk, or rosewater and glycerine cleansers everyday, and use any of the others occasionally to treat your skin to a special cleansing routine.

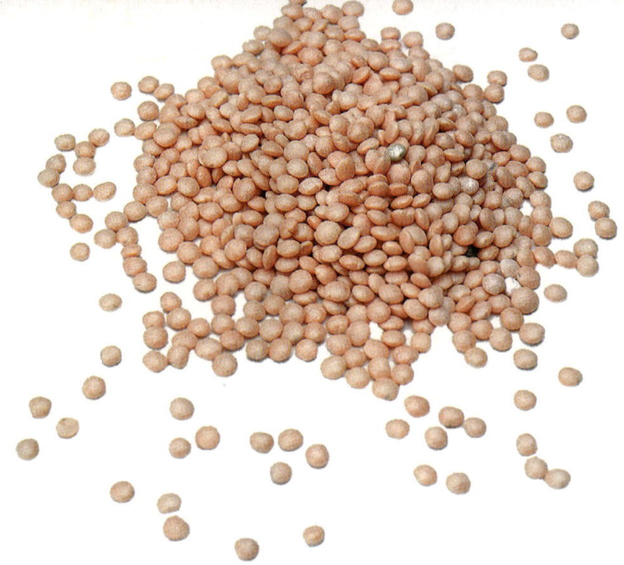

Rejuvenate with Exfoliates

Sometimes one needs a more exhaustive cleansing routine. These need not be a daily ritual, but they are required to rejuvenate your skin, more so, if one has skin problems. You also need to get rid of dead skin cells. For this you need to use exfoliates.

Exfoliation is important as it stimulates the skin, and helps to get rid of dead skin cells, leading to a clearer skin with fewer lines and wrinkles. A word of caution here, everything is good within limits. Many women believe that they shold exfoliate everyday. Be cautious. One should never over-exfoliate as that may damage blood vessels especially, the delicate skin area on the face. This can cause redness and inflammation. Your skin type determines how often you should exfoliate. Ideally speaking, it should be done once a week. Women who have abnormally oily skins and an acne problem can do so twice a week. Never more than that. In winters, exfoliate less often than in summers.

Basically there are two types of exfoliates — mechanical and chemical. Mechanical exfoliates involve using an abrasive sponge or loofah to physically buff the skin. Sometimes using these too harshly can harm your skin. Instead, you could use mechanical exfoliates made from grains, pulses or even vegetables. Chemical exfoliates are commercially marketed products which use beta hydroxy acids to remove dead skin cells. These should be used only when advised by a beautician or cosmetologist. For normal requirements it is best to use exfoliates made from natural substances.

OATMEAL : Take half cup oatmeal. Add to this half teaspoon salt, one teaspoon honey and just a little cold milk to make a rough thick paste. Apply all over the forehead, face and neck. When it begins to dry up, rub using brisk, firm movements. A good exfoliate for tough skins acts as an abrasive agents and helps in exfoliation.

WHEAT HUSK : The flaky powder left behind when wheat flour is made, is the best exfoliate. You could use wheat porridge grains also. Take half cup of wheat husk or porridge. Add to this one tablespoon honey and one tablespoon of milk. Make a thick paste. Apply all over the forehead, face and neck (avoid the eyes). Exfoliate gently with a loofah, or use strong circular motions with the hand, keep rubbing for 5 minutes. Wash off. The skin becomes clean, baby soft and glowing.

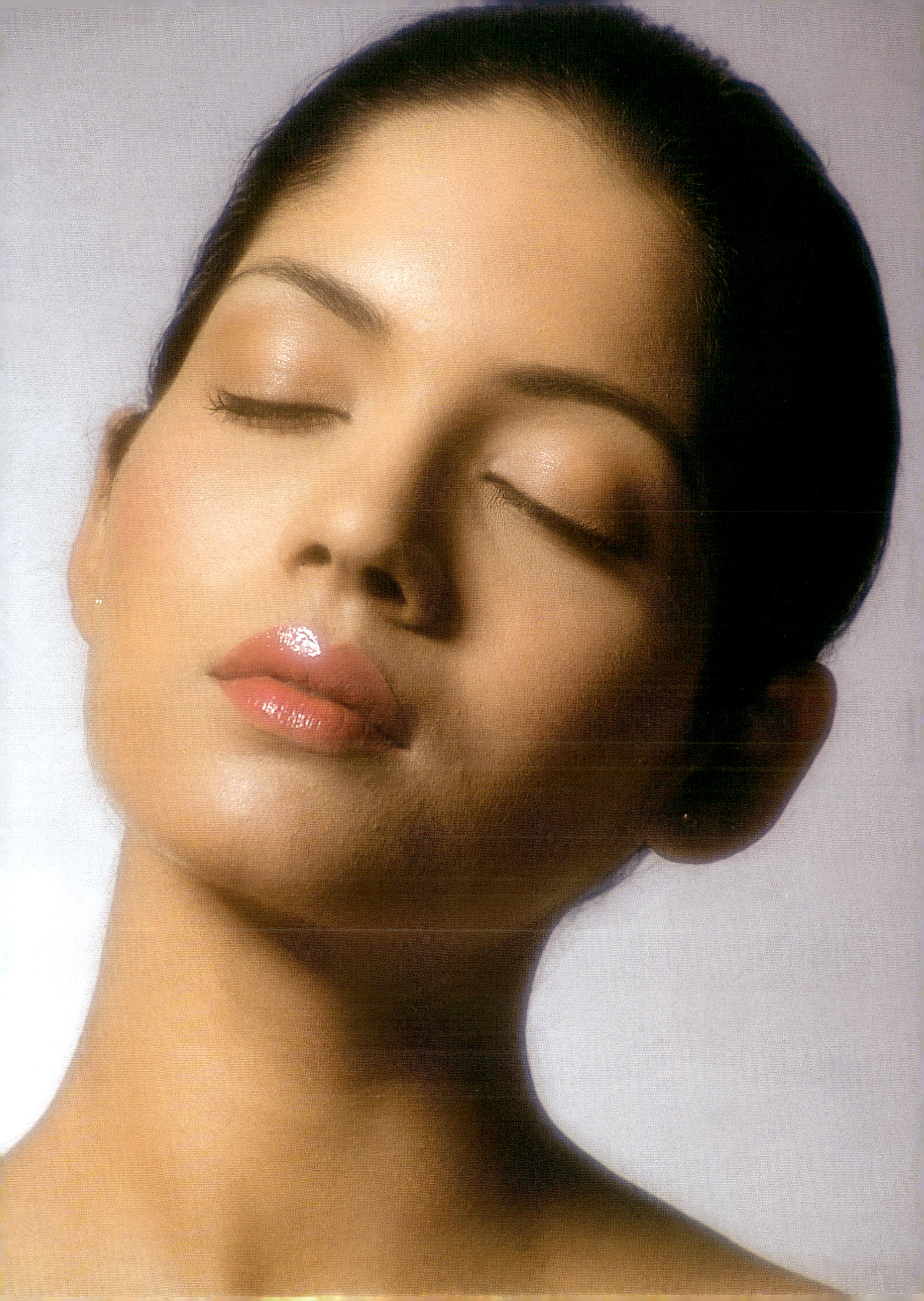

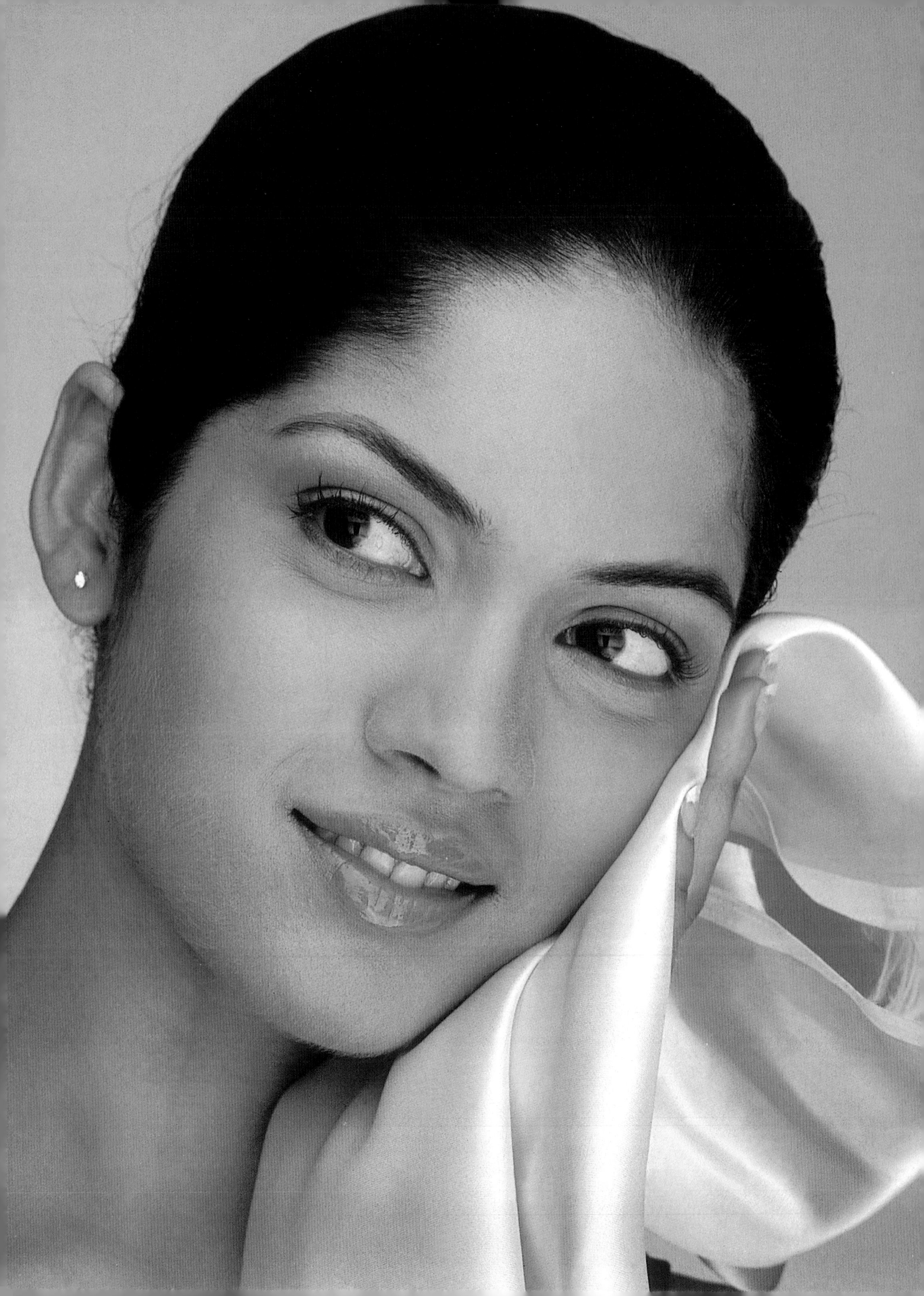

CHICKPEA POWDER : Take half cup chickpea powder. Add one teaspoon turmeric powder and one tablespoon olive oil (or any other oil like coconut). Mix and make a thick paste. Apply all over the forehead, face and neck (avoid the eyes).

When the paste starts to dry up, rub with your hands, scrubbing as you go along. Then wash it off with lukewarm water. This is a mild but effective exfoliate that also helps get rid of fine facial hair.

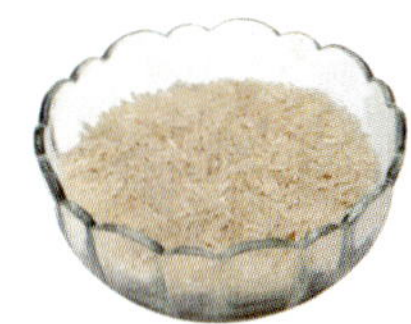

RICE : This makes an excellent exfoliate. Take half cup rice. Grind it coarsely to a powder. Add to it one tablespoon of honey and two tablespoons of beaten curd. Blend into a paste. Apply all over the forehead, face and neck. This paste dries up very fast, so rub quickly in circular motions. Scrub well and wash off.

YELLOW LENTIL : Take half cup of any yellow lentil. Soak for half an hour. Drain out the water. coarse grind it to a paste. Add to it a tablespoon of chickpea powder with just enough milk to make a thick paste. Apply all over the forehead, face and neck. Keep rubbing in circular motions to remove dead skin and clear blemishes. This is an ideal exfoliate for even very tender skin.

VEGETABLES : You can use cabbage leaves, the outer skin of sweet gourd, skin of tomato etc. Take grated cabbage leaves, tied in a thin piece of muslin and rub all over the forehead, face and neck. Keep rubbing, applying pressure. The same can be done with any other vegetable peels, or grated sweet gourd. These are the mildest of exfoliates and clean very gently.

Toners and Fresheners

Toners, fresheners and astringents belong to the same family. They help in smoothening your skin, and act as a balm after the exfoliation process. These help to seal skin pores, tighten the outer layers of the facial skin, also acting as a safety net after a heavy exfoliation and cleansing routine.

BERRIES : You could use strawberries, cherries, cranberries or blackberries to make this unique, rejuvenating toner and astringent at home.

Take one tablespoon honey, 2 tablespoons of pureed berries, one tablespoon oatmeal or wheat bran. Combine all the ingredients in a bowl.Wet your face. Apply this paste all over the forehead, face and neck (avoid the eyes). Let it remain for five minutes. Now gently rub it into your face. Rub and wash off with tepid water. The fruit acids in the berries shrink your pores, brighten up your face and tone your skin. Use this toner to really pamper yourself.

LIME : Take 2 cups of water. Add juice of two limes. To this solution add one tablespoon of tincture of benzoin as a preservative. Shake well and pour into a bottle and keep. Use this as an astringent. Very good for normal skin.

WATERCRESS : Take a handful of watercress salad leaves. Bruise them and add them to a saucepan containing equal parts of water and milk (one and a half cups should be enough). Simmer over a slow fire for a few minutes. Remove from the fire and mash the leaves well. Strain and pour the liquid into a bottle after cooling. Apply this lotion after a bath or after cleaning your face of all make-up. Let it dry on your face. This removes blemishes and gives the complexion a healing touch, making it soft and creamy. Wash off after 10–15 minutes.

CORNFLOWER : Take a handful of flowers and infuse in 250 ml of boiling water. Allow to cool. Mash the steamed flowers into the water. Add a teaspoon of which hazel (available at the chemist shop). Strain and pour into a bottle after cooling. An effective and soothing astringent.

ORANGE AND LEMON PEELS : Do not throw away orange and lemon peels. Sun dry them. When they are absolutely dry and brittle, powder them and keep them in a jar or wide mouthed bottle. This powder can be used in a number of face care preparations; as a moisturizing face pack, as an exfoliate and also as an astringent.

To use as an astringent, take 2 tablespoons of this powder, add to this 3 tablespoons of rosewater and 3 tablespoons of water. stir well and shake it up. Apply this lotion all over the forehead, face and neck. Be careful and avoid the eyes. Let it dry, then wash off. This is an excellent astringent that cures blemishes, shrinks open pores and a good cure for pimples.

CUCUMBER AND ROSEWATER : Take one cucumber. Peel and grate it. Take 3 tablespoons of rosewater and add the grated cucumber. Put it in a blender and make a paste and refrigerate. Use as a toner on dry sun-burnt skin. Apply all over; leave it on for 20 minutes. Rinse off. Excellent for sun burnt, dry skin.

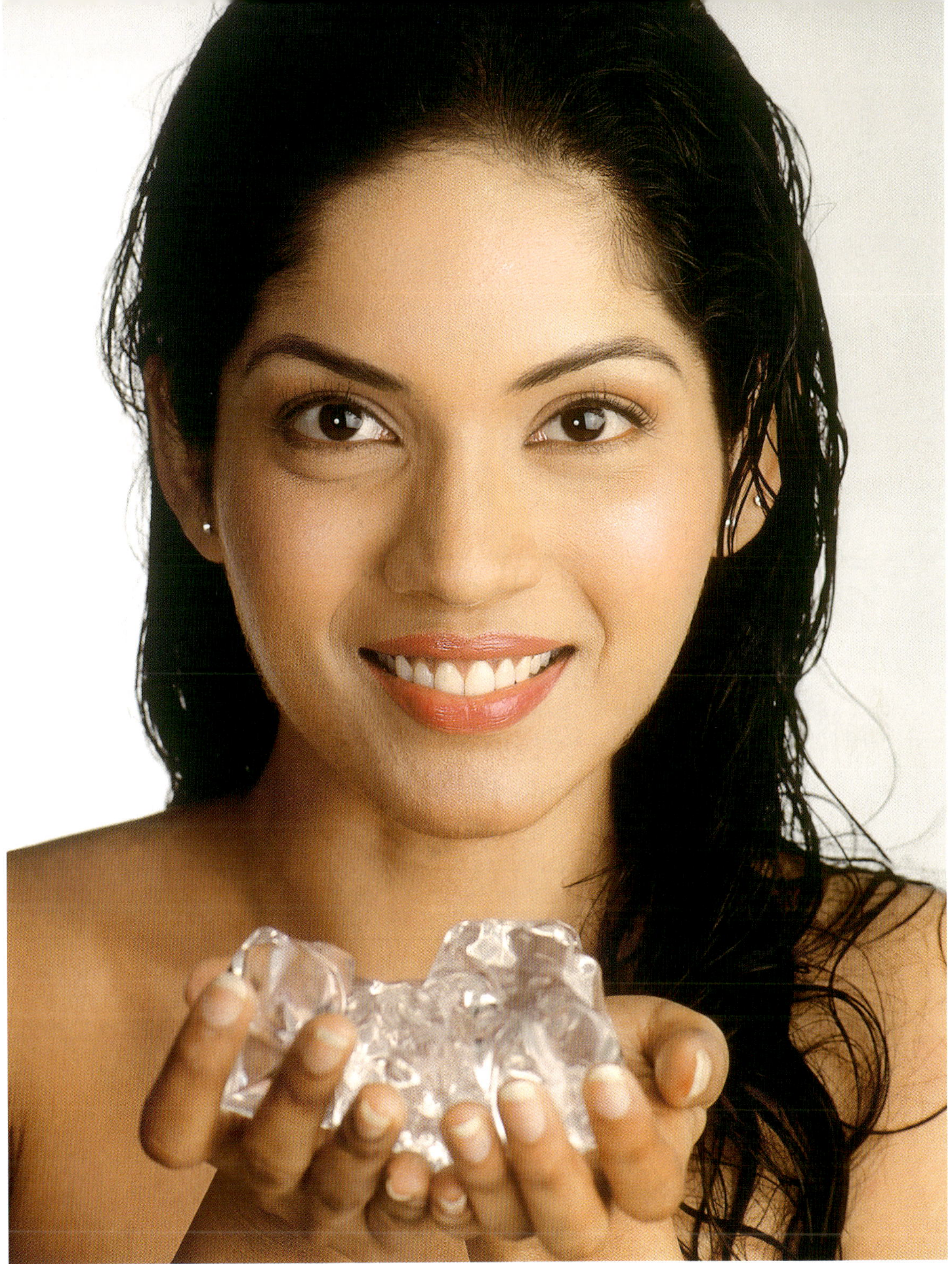

ICE CUBES : Take ice cubes and rub them all over the face. This tightens the pores and increases the blood circulation. An ideal, inexpensive and instant toner.

LEMON TREE FLOWERS : If you have a lime tree in your garden, you can make this effective complexion lotion. Take a handful of lemon flowers and infuse them in 20 ml of boiling water. Let it cool. Mash flowers and strain. To this add equal part of rose water. Pour in a bottle, refrigerate and keep. Use after a bath or after cleaning your face. Especially good after you apply at bedtime and leave it on overnight.

Moisturisers and Face Packs

A rigorous cleaning and exfoliating routine leaves the skin hungry for food and nourishment. You need a good moisturiser or face pack to nourish your skin. In fact you need to use moisturisers at least twice a day.

EGG AND ALMOND MOISTURISER : Take one egg yolk and add to it one tablespoon almond oil or take 5 almonds and crush them to a fine powder and then add to the egg yolk. Add one tablespoon of honey to this. Stir well and apply to the forehead, face and neck (avoid the eyes). Leave it on for 15 minutes. Rinse, first with warm water then with cold.

FULLER'S EARTH AND HONEY : Take 2 tablespoons of fuller's earth. Add to it one tablespoon of honey and one tablespoon of milk. Mix well. Apply this paste all over the forehead, face and neck (avoid the eyes). Leave it on for 15 minutes, and then wash off with cold water. The fuller's earth seals the pores while the honey and milk nourish the skin.

MARIGOLD FLOWERS : Take 2 cups of marigold petals. Soak them in a bowl of water and keep aside. After 2–3 hours, when the petals are limp, mash them well with your hands in the same water. To this paste add one tablespoon of glycerine. Mix well. Apply to the forehead, face and neck (avoid the eyes). Wash off after 10 minutes. An unusual, but very effective, skin tonic.

LEMON JELLY : Take a packet of lemon jelly and add to it a cup of boiling water. Stir and mix well, and add to this the juice of one lemon. Stir and let it set in the refrigerator. Just before using, steam your face to open up the pores. Apply chilled jelly to the forehead, face and neck (avoid the eyes). Leave it on for 15 minues then rinse off. This is an excellent cure for oily skin as lemon absorbs the excess oil from your skin.

PARSLEY : Take a handful of parsley. Chop it finely and put it in a bowl. Pour 2–3 tablespoons of boiling water over it. Add one tablespoon of light olive oil and mash well to make a thick paste. Apply to the forehead, face and neck (avoid the eyes). Leave it on for 5–10 minutes. Remove gently. Wash it off with warm water. Parsley has antibiotic properties that kills germs. The olive oil helps to shrink the pores. This pack is especially useful when you come back from a polluted environment. Useful for all skin types.

WATERMELON : There is no better method of refreshing the body and sun-scorched face than to use a watermelon. Watermelon instantly restores lost moisture, tightens the skin and leaves it looking fresh. It is also simple to use. Just cut slices of watermelon, squeeze some lime juice on them and apply to the forehead, face and neck (avoid the eyes). Keep rubbing in hard circular motions as you go along. Alternatively, you could puree the fruit, add lime juice and apply like a face pack. Leave it on for 20 minutes and wash it off. A squeaky clean, glowing skin emerges.

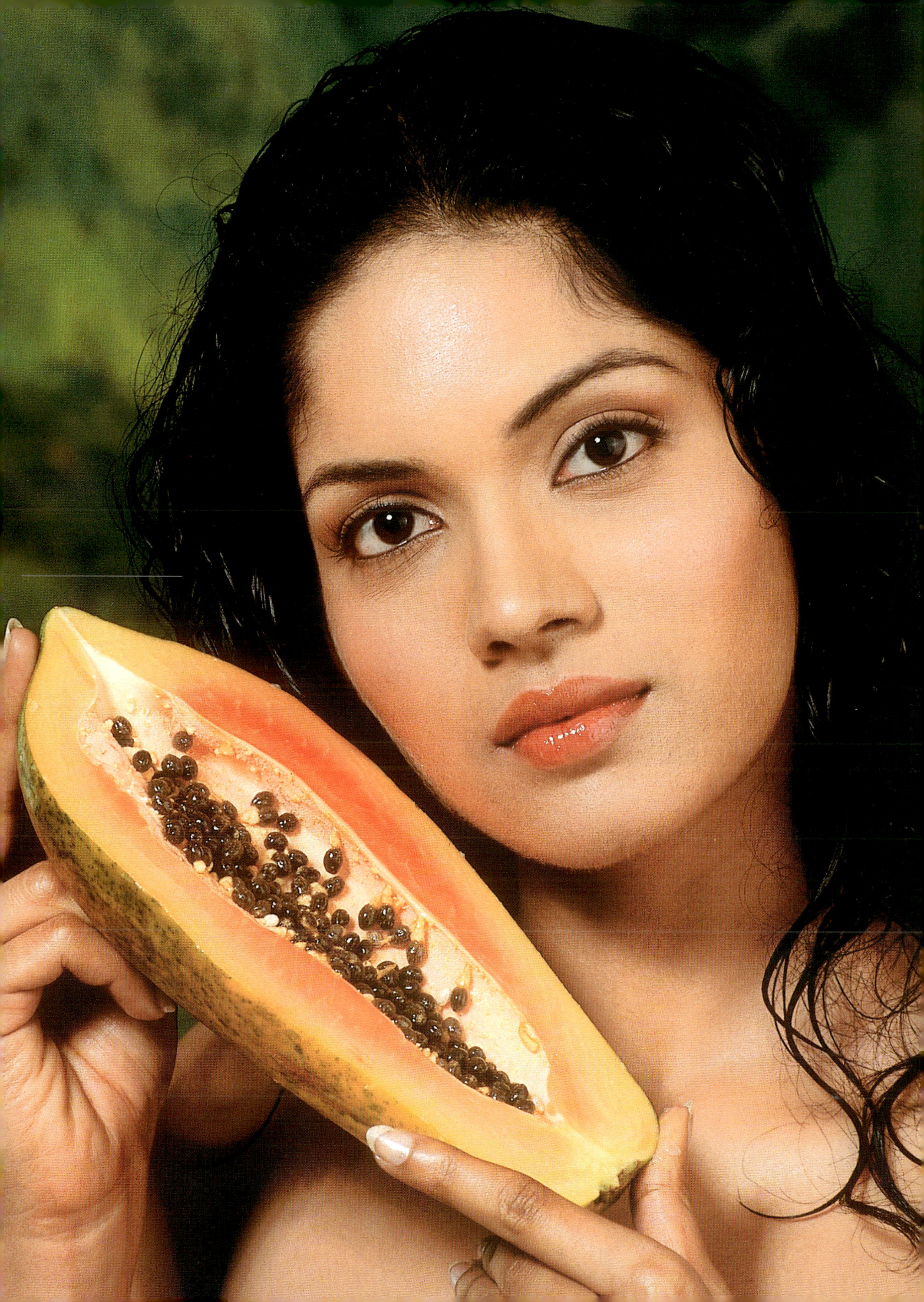

STRAWBERRIES : An excellent nourishment for people with oily skin. It feeds your skin yet, absorbs excess oil. Take a handful of strawberries, chop and put in blender. Add the juice of one lime and half cup yoghurt or cream and blend well. Pour in a container, refrigerate for 30 minutes and apply to the forehead, face and neck (avoid the eyes). When it begins to cake, apply again. Let it stand for 20 minutes, then rinse off by rubbing gently into the skin.

AVOCADO : Very popular with most beauticians, who make liberal use of this fruit for a variety of beauty treatments. Chop and put the fruit in a blender. Add one teaspoon honey, a little lemon juice and half cup yoghurt. Blend to make a thick paste. Pour into a jar and refrigerate for 30 minutes. Massage well into the face and neck. Wash off with plain water.

APRICOT : Another favourite with beauticians, also used in several beauty care products too. Take 2–3 apricots, de-seed them, chop and put them in a blender. Add to this half cup yoghurt or thick cream. Whip and pour into a container. Apply to the forehead, face and neck (avoid the eyes). When it starts caking, apply some more. Let it stand for 20 minutes, then wash off. It's an excellent nourishment for your skin.

PAPAYA : You can use the papaya fruit instead of the apricot to make a similar skin nourishment potion. Papaya effectively rejuvenates tired, jaded and dry skin. Regular use yields astonishing results.

ALMOND : Take 10–15 almonds and grind them finely. Take half cupful of yoghurt or sour cream. Add to it the almond powder and mix well to form a smooth paste. Apply to the forehead, face and neck (avoid the eyes). Leave it on for 20 minutes and then wash off. An excellent tonic for dry blemished skin.

OATS : Take a cupful of oatmeal. Add beaten yolks of 2 eggs and one tablespoon of honey. Add a few drops of tincture of benzin. Whip all this together in a bowl. Pour in a jar and keep in the refrigerator. You can use this several times. Take a little of this thick creamy paste and apply to the forehead, face and neck (avoid the eyes). Massage into the skin and leave it on for 15 minutes. Rinse off with lukewarm water.

ORANGE PEEL AND ROSEWATER : Take 3 tablespoons of dry orange peel powder and add to this a few dried powdered rose petals. Add one teaspoon of honey and just enough milk to form a thick paste. Apply to the forehead, face and neck (avoid the eyes). Let it stand for 20 minutes, then wash off. This unique moisturising pack leaves your skin as soft as a baby's skin.

You can certainly arrest ageing and keep your skin looking healthy by following these simple, yet, very effective face-care rituals and routines. This does not mean that there are no other skin problems that have to be dealt with. Pimples, pigmentation, dry skin, wrinkles, oily skin and blackheads are some of the common problems that women face. Given here are a few simple, easy to make cures for some. Patience is the keyword for effective treatment; the results will far exceed your expectations.

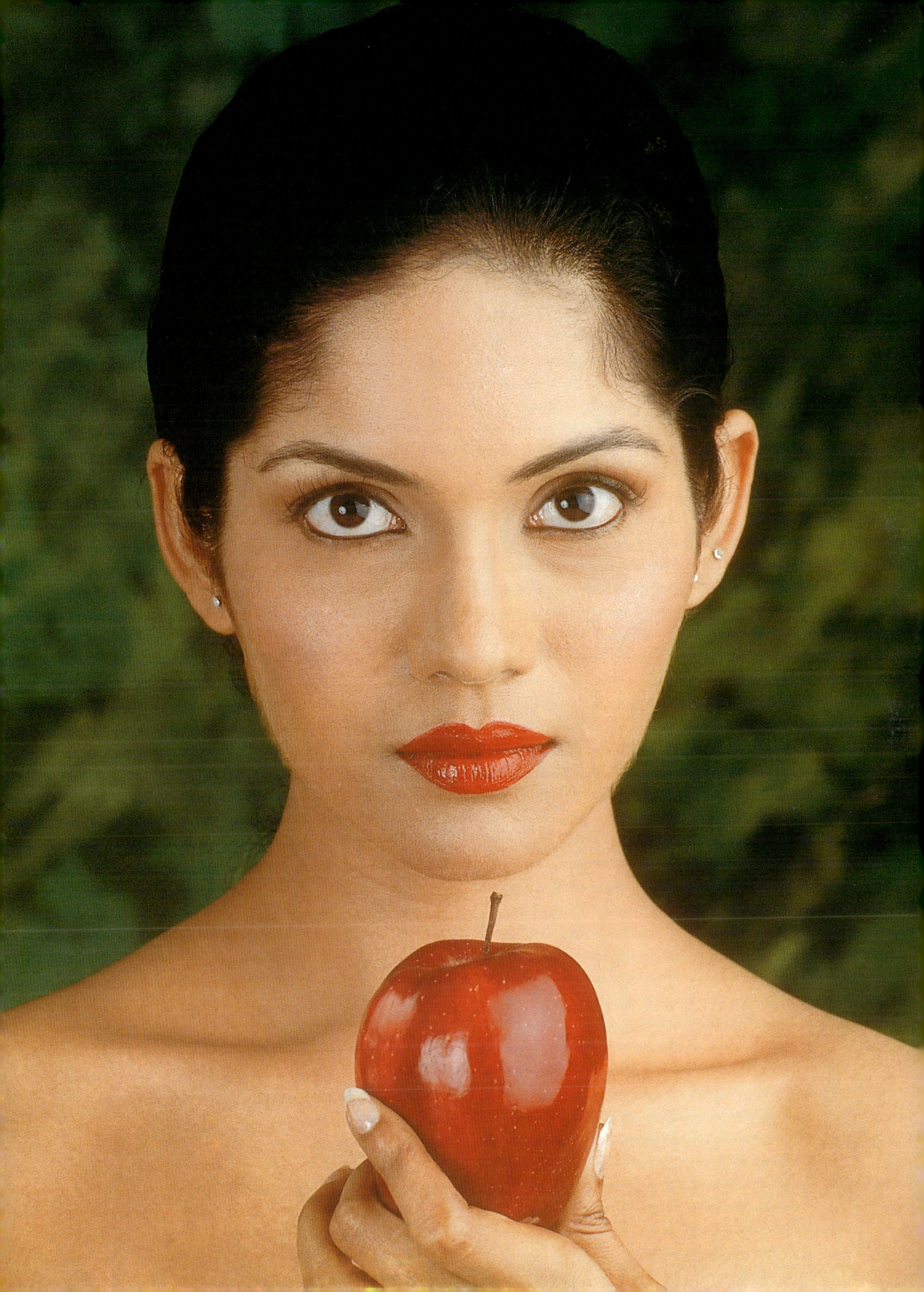

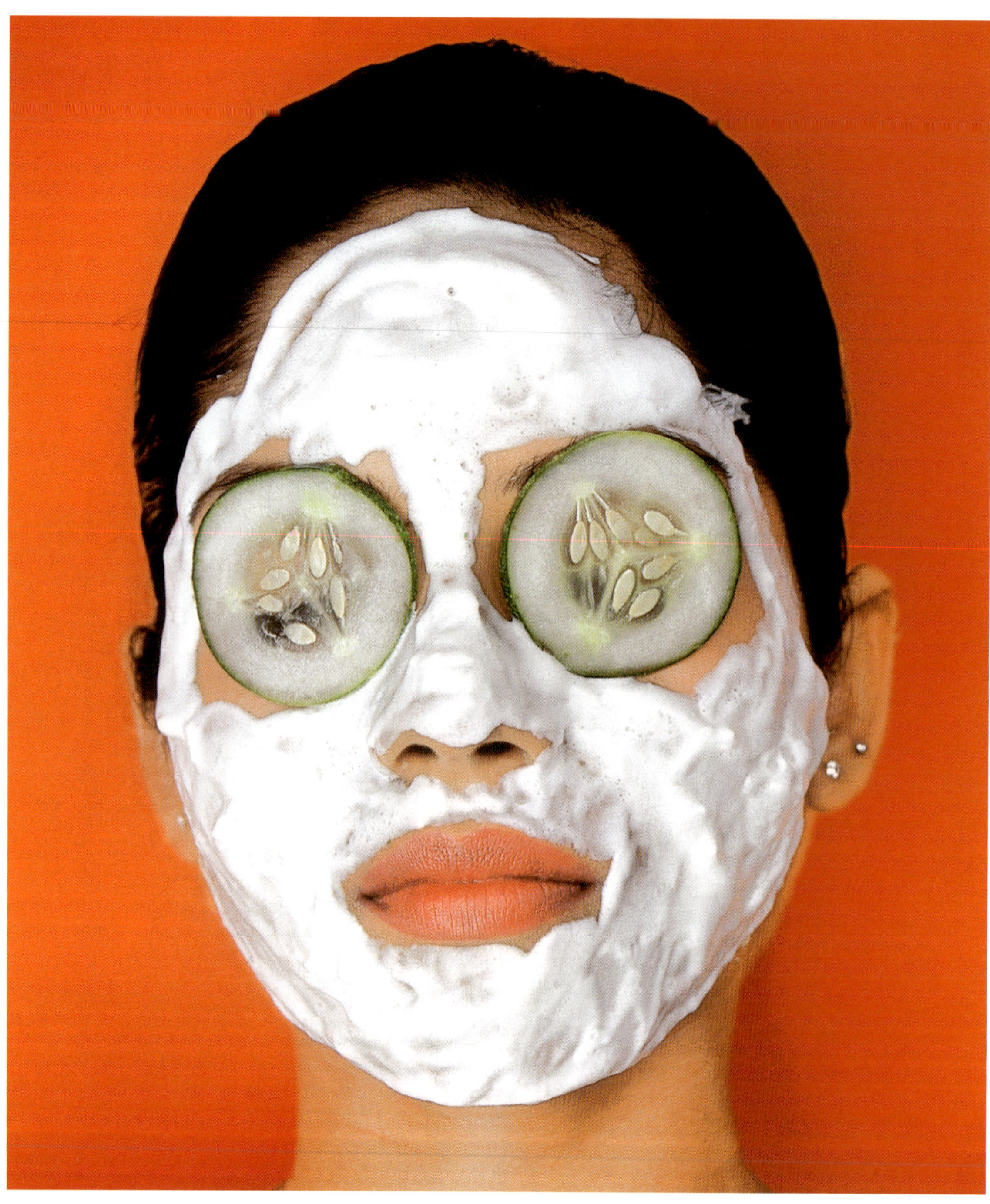

CARROT : Grate 2 carrots and add enough milk to make a thick, non-dripping paste. Spread it evenly all over the face, forehead and the neck. Leave it on for 20 minutes then wash off. This mask rejuvenates the skin.

Another very effective mask can be made with grated carrots and egg yolk. Add beaten egg yolk to the grated carrots and add one teaspoon of almond or olive oil. Mix well in a blender to form a smooth paste. Apply all over the forehead, face and neck. Leave it on for 15 minutes. Use cotton wool dipped in warm milk to wipe it off. Follow with a rinse.

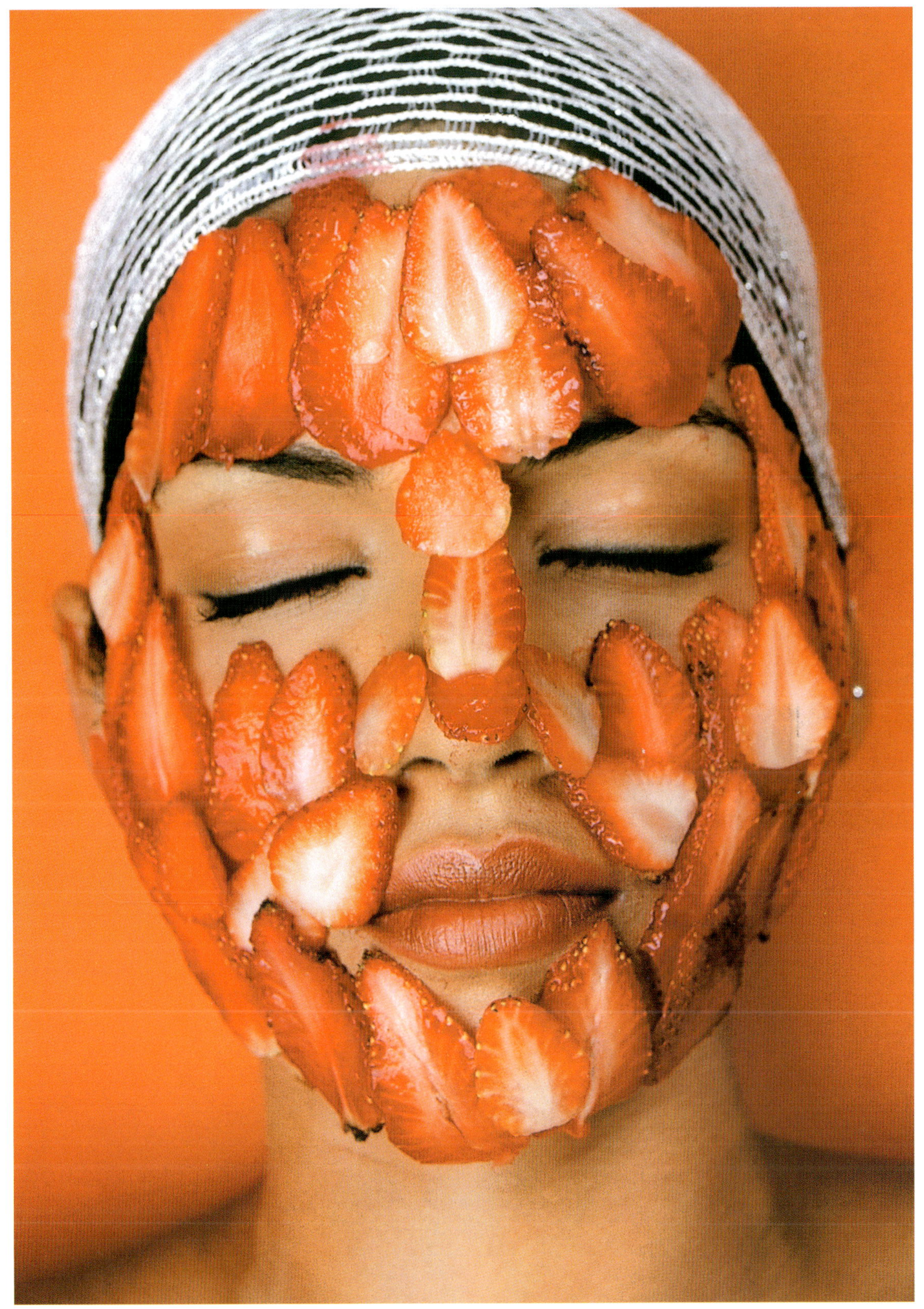

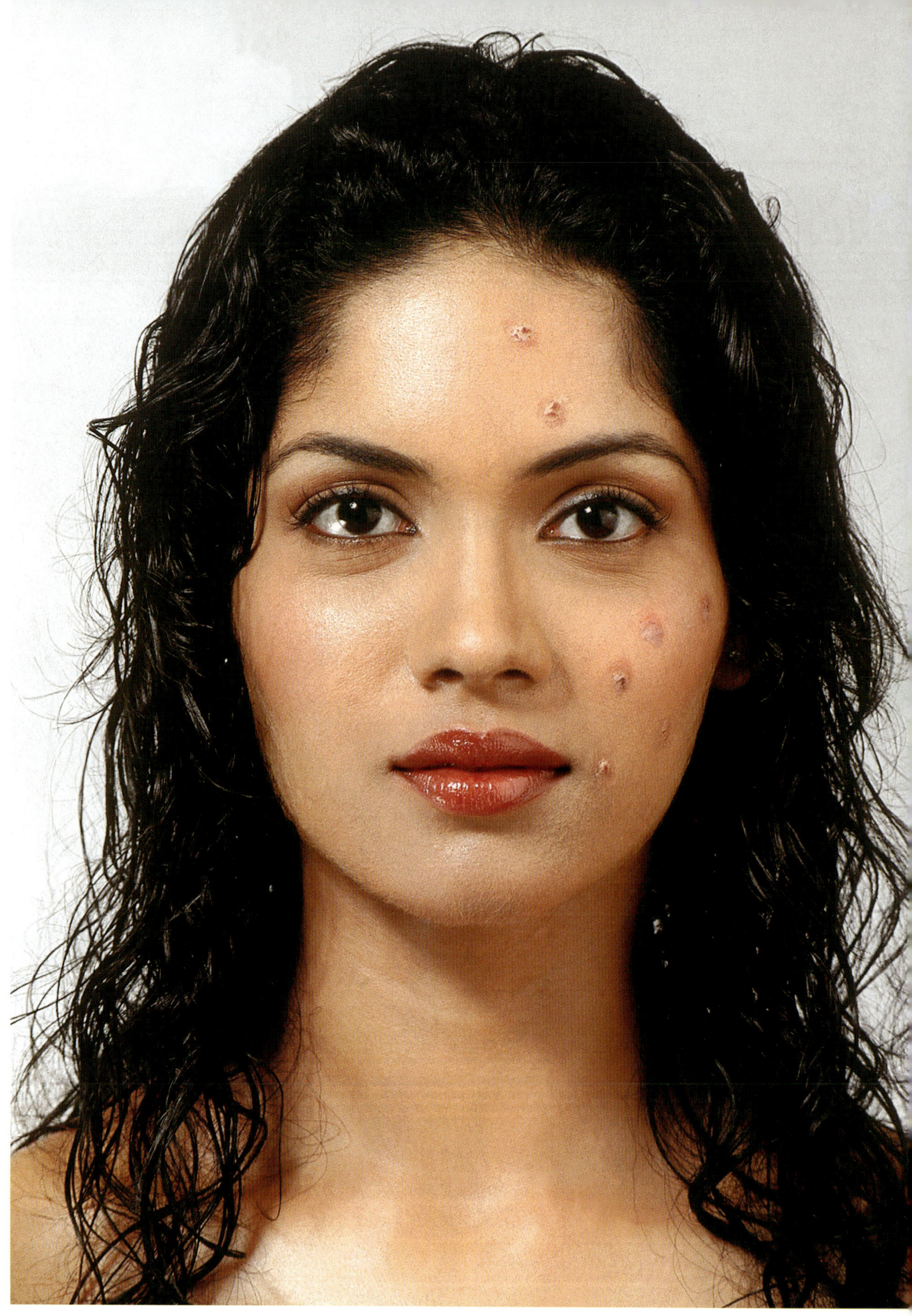

Growing Up With Acne

Every age has its own problems. Acne, pimples and blackheads are some of the common problems that cause anguish during the process of growing up.

Acne is mostly a problem of adolescence, though it could be due to hormonal imbalance too. The female hormones, estrogen and progesterone, are produced during the early growing up years, and the body needs time to adjust to this. An imbalance is created. The androgen hormones produced by the adrenal glands also affect the texture of the skin. The result of all these hormonal changes can manifest into excessive oiliness of the skin and scalp and also excessive perspiration. Too much secretion of oil clogs the pores, leading to blackheads and spots. Infected blackheads may lead to acne and pimples. A very aggressive cleanliness regime is needed to combat this situation. A few simple Do's and Don'ts will help.

Don't ever "pick" a pimple. The natural healing cycle for a pimple is 7 days. According to dermatologists, when you "pick" a pimple, you interrupt this cycle and set back the healing process by another 7 days. The best thing is to wait and let it dry on its own.

DO'S

- Drink lots of water.
- Clean your face as often as you can.
- Use astringents to help get rid of excess oil.
- Eat more fruits and raw vegetables.
- Bathe frequently and use cooling lotions during summer.
- Keep your nails trimmed neatly to avoid dirt being carried to your face and increase chances of infection.

DON'T

- Eat oily and starchy foods.
- Use any make-up.

Blackheads, acne and pimples can indeed be controlled with the help of ingredients from your kitchen. A word of caution. If your infection is mild, then these simple remedies along with a controlled diet will suffice. However for major infections it is best to take the doctor's advice too.

BLACK PEPPER AND CURD : Take one tablespoon black pepper powder and add to it enough curd to make a thick paste. Apply on the infected area and let it dry. Wash off after 5–7 minutes. This is an effective cure for blackheads.

OATMEAL AND YOGHURT : Take 2 tablespoons of oatmeal and 3 tablespoons of yoghurt. Mix and add one tablespoon of lemon juice and one teaspoon of olive oil. Blend and whisk well together in a bowl. Wash your hands and then apply over infected area first, then all over the face. Leave on for 5–7 minutes and then rinse with cold water. Very effective for blackheads.

TOMATO JUICE : Normally, pimples and acne are associated with an oily skin. In case these occur on a dry skin then this is the ideal treatment. Take a few tomatoes and puree them. Freeze the puree into cubes (in an ice cube tray). Store these frozen tomato ice cubes in a bag or a container in the freezer. During the day, apply one cube each on either cheek, all the time rubbing gently. Repeat the treatment everday. A very effective way of getting rid of pimples.

ALMOND, LEMON AND OLIVE OIL : Powder 10 almonds and add to this the juice of 2 lemons. Add 2 tablespoons of olive oil, mix well and store. Keep in a jar and use twice a day. Its helps in curing pimples.

POTATO AND MILK : Pimples leave behind an ugly scar when they dry and fall off. To get rid of these scars use this and see the results. Take 2 potatoes. Skin and grate them. Extract the juice and to this add 2–3 tablespoons of cold milk. Stir well and apply all over the pimple scars. Let it dry and gently rub and wash off. Use this treatment regularly, at least twice a day.

ORANGE PEEL AND YOGHURT : An ideal mask that extracts dirt and oil from clogged pores. It also opens up the clogged pores that cause acne and blackheads. Take 2 tablespoons of orange peel powder and add 4 tablespoons of yoghurt to make a paste. Apply all over the face, while gently rubbing in circular motion. Wash off with cold water. An excellent way to prevent clogged pores and keep the skin clean and healthy.

APPLE JUICE : Take an apple, peel and grate it to extract the juice. Add one teaspoon of honey and apply on face. Dab gently on the pimples and let it dry. Apply again. Repeat this treatment at least twice a day. Your pimples will dry and the scars will vanish with regular treatment.

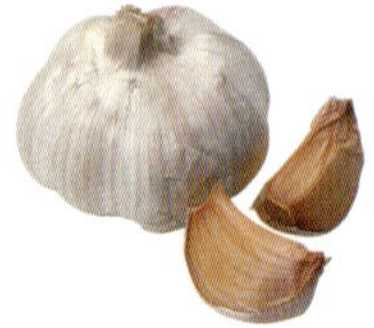

GARLIC : Take a few pods of garlic and crush them fine. Add a few drops of honey and add some curd to make a paste. Apply gently only on the pimples. Let it dry, and then wash gently without scrubbing. Regular use helps dry the pimples faster and healing is much quicker. Be careful to use this paste only on the pimples.

TOMATO AND YOGHURT : Take 2/3 tablespoons of tomato puree and add a little beaten yoghurt. Also add one tablespoon boiled oatmeal paste or boiled porridge. Blend all these into a paste. Apply all over the face and let it dry. Rinse with cold water. An effective way to rid yourself of pimples.

MINT : Take a few mint leaves and crush them finely. Tie them in a piece of muslin and squeeze it to extract the juice. Apply the juice all over the face. Dab gently with cotton wool pads on the pimples. Wash off and use at least once a week. It controls pimples.

FULLER'S EARTH AND ROSEWATER : This makes an ideal acne pack for oily skin. Take 2 tablespoons of fuller's earth and add one tablespoon of rosewater and 2 tablespoons of curd. Mix all these to form a thick paste. Apply this on the face and leave it for 20 minutes, and then wash it off. Regular use once a week is good for mild acne problems.

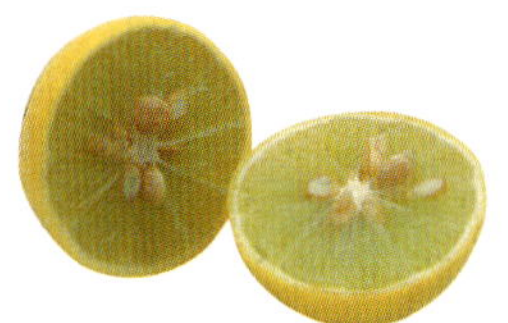

EAU DE COLOGNE AND LEMON JUICE : Mix an equal quantity of eau de cologne with boiled and cooled lemon juice. Apply this solution on the pimples. Leave to dry and then apply again. Wash off after the application has dried. Repeat the treatment at night. This helps in drying the pimples faster.

CLOVES : Take a few pods of cloves and roast them dry in a pan. Powder them and add a little curd to make a paste. Dab the paste on the pimples and let it dry. Wash off. Use this treatment regularly if you are prone to pimples. It is especially good for people who have an oily skin. The roasted cloves help to dry up the pimples faster.

TEA BAGS : Saturate 2 tea bags in warm water. Now press the wet tea bags onto the pimples. Press, dab 2 or 3 times on pimples and leave it to dry. Rinse after a while.

A few handy tips for those who suffer from pimple 'attacks'. Drink plenty of water and vegetable or fruit juices. Use cucumber or other fruit and vegetable packs to cure pimple scars. Maintain a diet that is rich in cottage cheese, fish and yoghurt. These help to cleanse your system and ward off pimples.

Every morning the first thing you should have is a glass of carrot juice or a glass of lime juice with honey. These are excellent 'tonics' to cleanse your system and help in giving you a clean, glowing complexion.

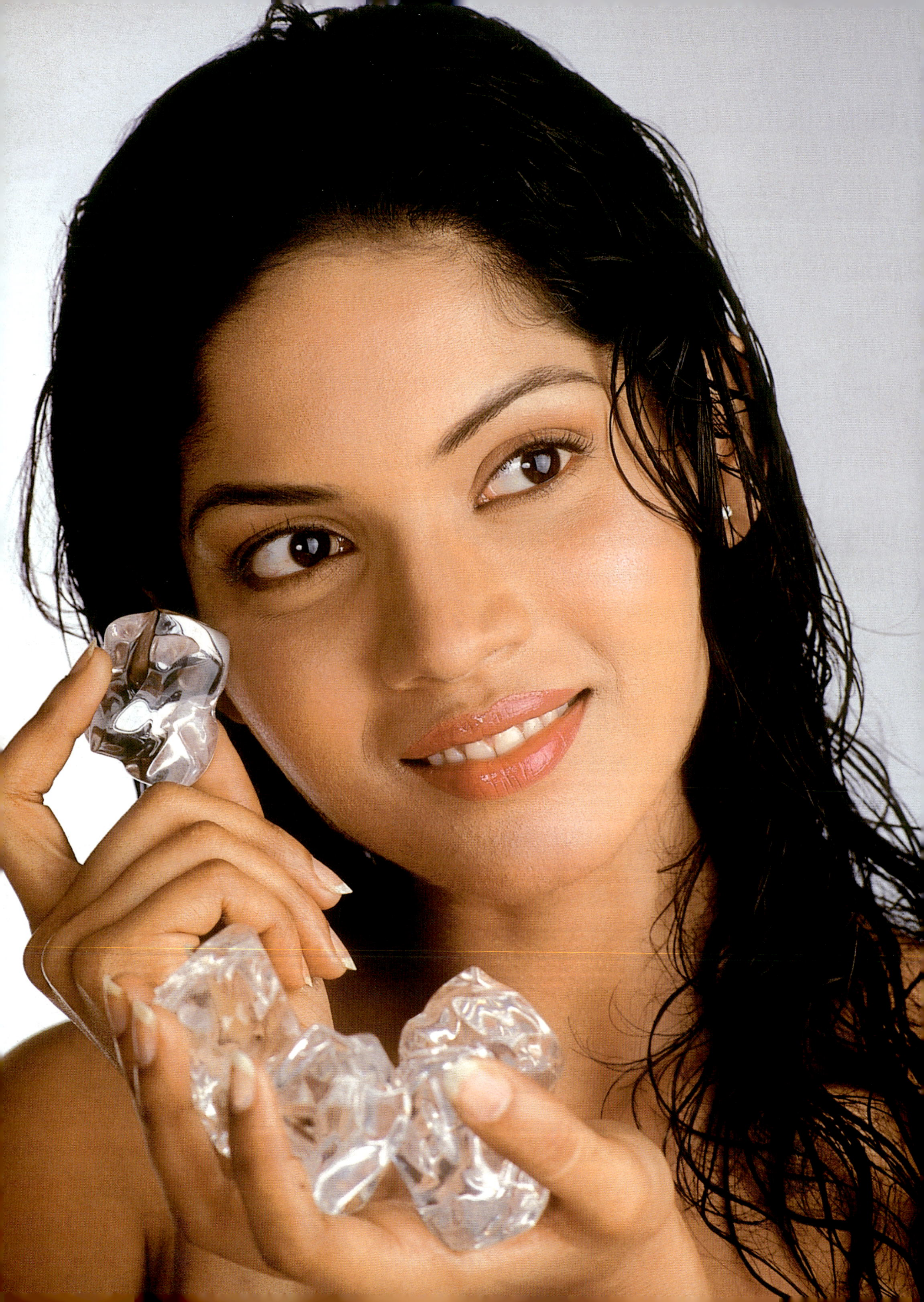

Blemishes, Shadows and Scars

Exposure to the sun and the vagaries of nature lead to different reactions on the skin. Some people get scars and blemishes while others suffer from sunburn and tan. A few precautionary measures and regular application of useful remedies would certainly help you combat these problems.

UNDER-EYE SHADOWS

These are usually caused by tension and tiredness of the eyes. Overwork, long hours of exposure of work at a computer screen, lack of sleep and of course ageing process - all contribute to this problem. One tends to rush and buy the latest 'under-eye' cream. A word of caution here, some of them may be too rich and extra moisturising and could result in causing puffiness in the under-eye area. Always use a light moisture-based cream. To cure these problems at home use the following:

CUCUMBER : Clean your face of all makeup. Cut out thin slices of cucumber. Chill them. Now lie down and shut your eyes. Apply chilled cucumber slices over your eyes and under-eye area and relax. Leave it on for 15 minutes. Gently rub the slices over the eyes and under-eye areas, and then wash off. You will feel relaxed and refreshed. The natural moisture from the cucumber acts as a healing tonic, while the cucumber juice helps to lighten the skin too. A great relief for tired and puffy eyes.

ICE CUBES : When you get in from the hot sun your eyes get tired and bloodshot. You also develop dark circles and shadows due to the heat and pollution. Try this: wash your face. Take some ice cubes and wrap them in two pieces of muslin. Lie down and shut your eyes. Place one ice cube pack over each eye, rubbing gently. This will immediaely ease the 'burnt up skin' feeling. Regular use helps to lighten the shadows under the eyes.

GREEN GOURD : You could similarly use slices of green gourd instead of cucumber. The juice of the green gourd also helps in lightly moisturizing as well as lightening the skin tones.

PATCHES ON THE FACE

Sometimes due to hormonal changes, lack of proper nourishment or even due to stress, your facial skin becomes patchy—light in certain areas and dark in others. Use the following to get rid of patches as well as shadows and 'brown' spots.

FULLER'S EARTH AND LIME : Take one tablespoon fuller's earth, add one teaspoon of lime juice and enough rosewater to make a smooth paste. Apply this paste all over the face, rubbing it in gently. Leave it to dry and then apply again on the dark patches or spots. Leave it on for a further 5–7 minutes then wash and rinse with cold water. Use this treatment everyday to get rid of the patches.

MINT JUICE : Take a few mint leaves and crush them. Tie in a piece of muslin and extract its juice. Use this pure mint juice all over the face. Excellent for spots and blemishes.

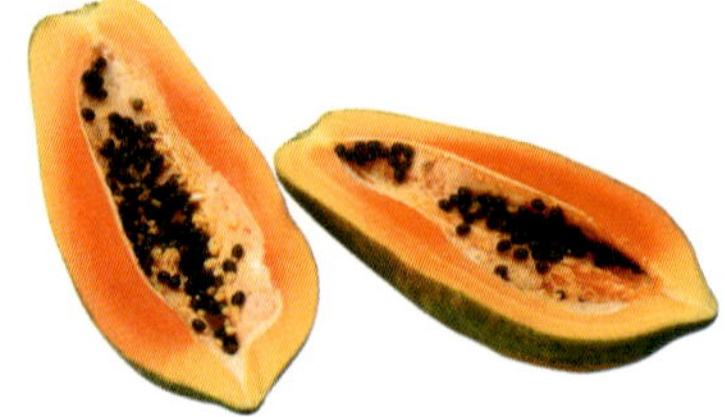

PAPAYA PACK : Take 2–3 slices of a ripe papaya and extract the pulp. Add to it one teaspoon of turmeric powder and one tablespoon of fuller's earth. Mash together to form a paste. Apply generously on the patches and dark areas of the skin. Leave it to dry. Then rinse it off. Regular use, maybe thrice a week, helps to even out the patches and blemishes.

CUCUMBER AND LIME JUICE : Take a cucumber and grate it after peeling. To this add juice of one lime. Mix well and put it into a blender to make a fine paste. Apply this paste all over the face and let it dry. Wash off. Regular use lightens shadows and scars.

VINEGAR AND ROSEWATER : Take 2 tablespoons of vinegar and add one tablespoon of rosewater. Now add the juice of one cucumber. Stir well to form a lotion. Dab this lotion all over the face and let it dry. Repeat this procedure twice or thrice till the complete lotion has been used up. Helps to remove spots and blemishes if used regularly.

FULLER'S EARTH AND CAMPHOR : Take one tablespoon of fuller's earth and add to it half teaspoon camphor powder and one tablespoon lime juice. Blend well to form a smooth paste. Apply all over the face, rubbing it in gently. Leave it to dry. Rinse and wash off.

CARROT PACK : Take 2–3 carrots and grate them after peeling. Boil the grated carrots in very little water till the water dries up. Cool and mash. Apply this pack all over the face. Leave it on for 10–15 minutes; gently rub it in before rinsing off.

BANANA PACK : An ideal 'food' for the face. It not only nourishes the skin but also 'magically' removes scars, dark patches and blemishes. You will notice the change even after using this once. Take a ripe banana, peel and mash to a pulp. Apply al over the face and leave it on for 10 minutes. Wash off and see your skin come out sparkling clean and nourished.

POTATO PACK : Take a raw potato, peel and grate it. Put the grated potato into a muslin piece and tie it tightly to form a pad. Rub this pad all over the face in firm, circular motions for about 5 minutes and then wash your face. Alternatively you could directly rub potato slices all over your face. Helps to clear blemishes and scars.

COCONUT OIL AND CAMPHOR : In case of minor burns that leave scars, this is a good recipe. Take 2 tablespoons of coconut oil and add to it one teaspoon of camphor powder. Rub thoroughly into the burn mark or scar at least 10 minutes before your bath. Use regularly for quick results.

There will be a marked lightening of the scar after a few days.

DRIED ORANGE PEELS : Take a few dried orange peels and powder them. Add 2 tablespoons of curd to make a thick paste. Apply all over the face, leaving aside the eye area. Let it dry, then wash thoroughly with cold water. Helps remove blemishes and scars.

FRECKLES

Unevenly distributed melanin (pigmentation) occurs due to exposure to the sun. People who have a fine textured skin and a fair complexion usually get freckles. You should not get unduly upset. Never try and cover up the freckles with makeup, that will only make matters worse. You should rather to lighten them.

LEMON, ORANGE OR LIME JUICE : The juice of any one of these can be mixed with a little beaten yoghurt. This paste should be regularly applied on the face and left to dry. Rinse off with cold water. This will help to lighten the freckles.

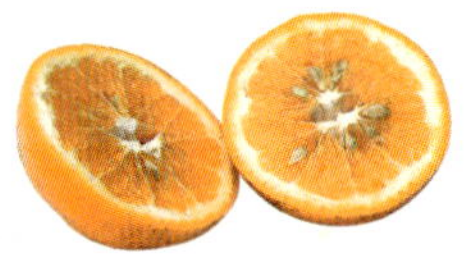

RADISH : Radish contains a bleaching agent. So take one radish, grate it and add to it the juice of one lime. Blend well and apply all over the face. Leave to dry and then wash off. It not only lightens the freckles but also removes blackheads. Rub vigorously before washing to remove the blackheads.

MINT AND BANANA : Take a few mint leaves and grind them to a paste. Add to this one mashed banana and blend in a blender. Apply this paste all over the face — be careful to avoid the eyes. Regular use will lighten the freckles and remove blemishes too.

EGGPLANT : Take an eggplant and slice it. Apply fresh eggplant slices all over the freckles, keep rubbing them in a circular motion and leave them on for a few minutes. Use this treatment daily and the results will show after a week.

CRANBERRY AND STRAWBERRY : Rub freshly crushed cranberries or strawberries on your face. Leave the juices and the mashed fruit on your face to dry. Then rinse with cold water. Regular use will lighten the freckles.

LEMON JUICE AND BORIC ACID : Dissolve one teaspoon boric acid in a cupful of hot water, and add to it the juice of one lemon. Add 2 tablespoons of rose water and half tablespoon of glycerine. Mix well and store this solution in a jar. Dab this lotion on the freckles with a cotton wool pad. Leave it on and later, rinse with water. Regular use will lighten the freckles. If the same solution in rubbed on the neck and shoulders, it makes them fairer, as they usually appear darker than the face.

SUNBURN AND TAN

Having a clear, glowing suntanned skin is the desire of most women. True, the rays of the sun are an essential revitaliser, they are good for the body as they help in the formation of vitamin D; however, over-exposure to the rays of the sun can also lead to many problems. It can cause sunburn, redness, sores and even blistering. Thus, some people with delicate skin types need to use a good and effective suntan oil. In cases of over-exposure, tanning and sunburn, here are a few excellent remedies.

CUCUMBER AND MILK : Take a cucumber, skin it and chop it finely and put it in a blender. Make a puree and add one tablespoon of chilled milk. Mix well and apply all over the face, neck, arms and areas scorched or burnt by the sun. Leave on for 15 minutes, and then rinse with cold water. Repeat this treatment twice or thrice during the course of the day. Its soothes the skin and helps in alleviating sunburn.

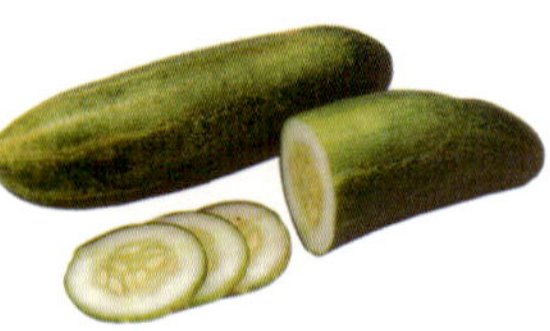

VINEGAR AND WATER : Take 2 tablespoons vinegar and add 2 tablespoons of water. This solution is an ideal cure for suntan. Dab on gently with cotton wool over sore areas. Leave it on for 10 minutes and wash off.

ONION : Take 2 onions, skin and chop them fine. Put then in a mixer and grind to a paste. Tie this in a muslin cloth and squeeze out the juice. Add to the juice a pinch of salt and a tablespoon of milk. Take cotton wool pads and dab over the sunburned or tanned areas. Leave to dry. Dab the juice again and repeat till the complete solution is used up. Let it dry on your skin. Rinse with cold water. It's best that you make it a routine after coming in from the hot sun.

CUCUMBER AND TOMATO WRAP : Take 2 tomatoes, puree them. Take a cucumber, peel and puree them too. Mix the purees and add to it the juice of one lemon. Mix well. Apply this paste all over the suntanned and sunburnt skin. Let it dry. Dab the puree again. Repeat 3 times and let it dry thoroughly, then rinse off. Use this treatment for a week and see the difference. It not only helps to soothe the burnt area, it adds a glow to the skin too.

CABBAGE : Take a handful of cabbage leaves, boil them and drain out the water. Mash the leaves and apply the pulp all over the tanned and sunburnt areas. Leave on for 15 minutes. Wash off with cold water. Repeat this treatment at least for a week. This acts like a protective and soothing balm. Use whenever you have been exposed to the hot sun.

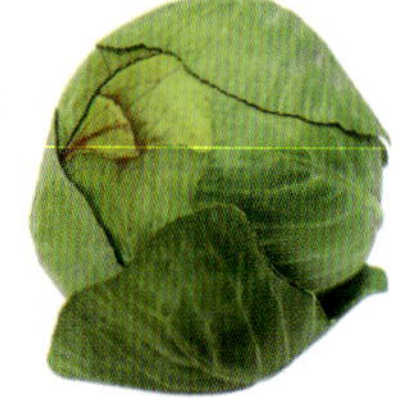

GREEN GOURD : Cut green gourd into thin round slices. Rub quickly all over the affected areas. Repeat 3–4 times. Leave it on and wash off at bedtime. Soothes burnt skin.

ALOE VERA : The most natural and soothing cure for sunburn and tan. Just pluck a few leaves of the plant, mash or puree them. Add the juice of one lemon. Apply this jelly like solution all over the affected areas. It cleanses, clears and nourishes the skin.

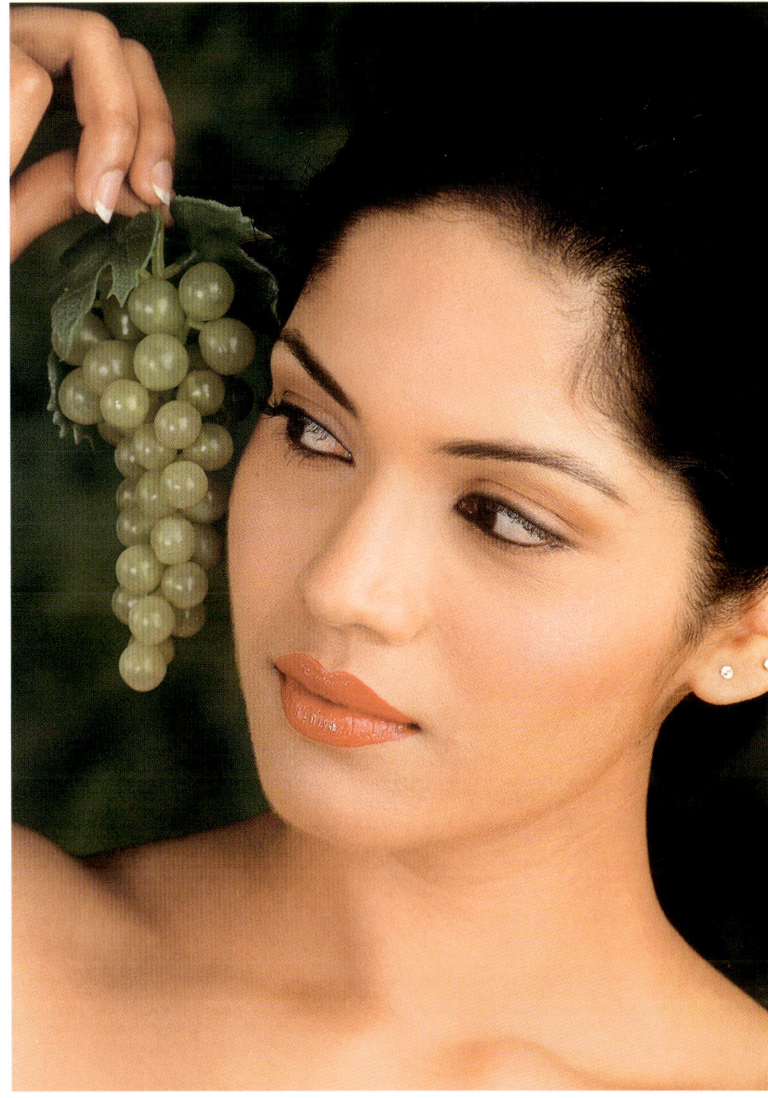

ICE : Use ice cubes all over the sunburned skin when you come from the hot sun.

HONEY AND LIME : Take 2 tablespoons of honey and add to it the juice of one lime. Mix well apply over the sunburned or tanned skin areas. Helps to lighten and soothe the skin.

LEMON AND SUGAR : Take the juice of one lemon and add to it a few grains of sugar. Rub this lotion all over the sunburned or tanned areas. Keep rubbing in circular motions. Let it dry and then wash off. This not only helps to remove tan but exfoliates the skin very gently too.

TUMERIC POWDER AND MILK Take 3 tablespoons of milk and add to it one tablespoon of turmeric powder. Apply all over the face or affected areas. Leave it to dry. Rub in circular motions and then rinse off. It not only helps to remove tan it also helps remove fine facial hair.

TOMATO AND OATMEAL : Puree 2 tomatoes. Add 2 tablespoons of curd and one tablespoon of oatmeal or wheat porridge. Mix to a smooth paste. Apply all over suntanned or sunburnt skin. Leave it on for 20 minutes and wash off with cold water. Helps in exfoliation too.

Wrinkles

An ageing skin requires a lot of care, a proper diet and a good exercise regimen to retain youthfulness. Women all over the world fear the onset of wrinkles. They go to extreme lengths to try and hide, camouflage and delay the process.

Thankfully, there are several natural cures. A proper diet of vegetables, fruits and herbs along with skin-nourishing cures not only delay wrinkles but also improve the texture of your skin. The use of such natural products does not lead to any side effects.

A word of caution too. Your attitude also determines how and when you get wrinkles. Frowning, knitting of the eyebrows, getting easily agitated causes the facial muscles to get tense and knotted up. This too contributes to early wrinkling. Cheer up, there are several simple cures that help. Smiling helps you relax your muscles too.

An ageing skin should take in plenty of fresh fruits and raw salads and yoghurt. The intake of liquids and water should increase manifold. We generally do not drink enough water.

YOGHURT AND CHICKPEA POWDER : Take half cup yoghurt and add 2 tablespoons of chickpea powder. Stir to a smooth paste. Apply a thick coat all over the face and neck. Let it stand for 10 minutes. Wash off. Repeat this every alternate day. This helps to tighten and nourish the skin.

APPLE : If you can use green apples there's nothing better. However any types of apples will also work wonders. De-seed and then puree an apple along with its skin. Add one tablespoon of milk and blend well. Apply this apple paste all over the face and neck. Keep taking more of the paste and massage well into the wrinkles. When it begins to dry up, rinse it off.

GLYCERINE AND EGG: This is an effective and an ideal anti-wrinkle lotion. Especially good for wrinkles on the hands and the neck. Take the white of an egg in a bowl and add to it 2 tablespoons of glycerine and 2 tablespoons of rose water. Stir well and then apply this lotion on the wrinkled skin as well as on the neck. Sit still and leave it on for 10–12 minutes. Rinse and wash off with cold water. An ideal application.

HONEY : Honey works like magic too. A mature skin that has been exposed to the sun and the wind can greatly benefit with this cure. Take 2 tablespoons of honey and to it, add the juice of an orange. Mix well and spread this all over your face and neck. Leave it on for 20 minutes. Gently wipe off with cotton wool dipped in milk. Use this treatment once a day, preferably at bedtime.

CABBAGE : Take enough cabbage leaves to give you half cup of cabbage juice extract. Add half teaspoon of wet yeast and one tablespoon of honey. Stir to a smooth paste and apply to the face and the neck. Sit still and relax, without making any facial movements. Let the paste dry up. When dry, wash off with lukewarm water.

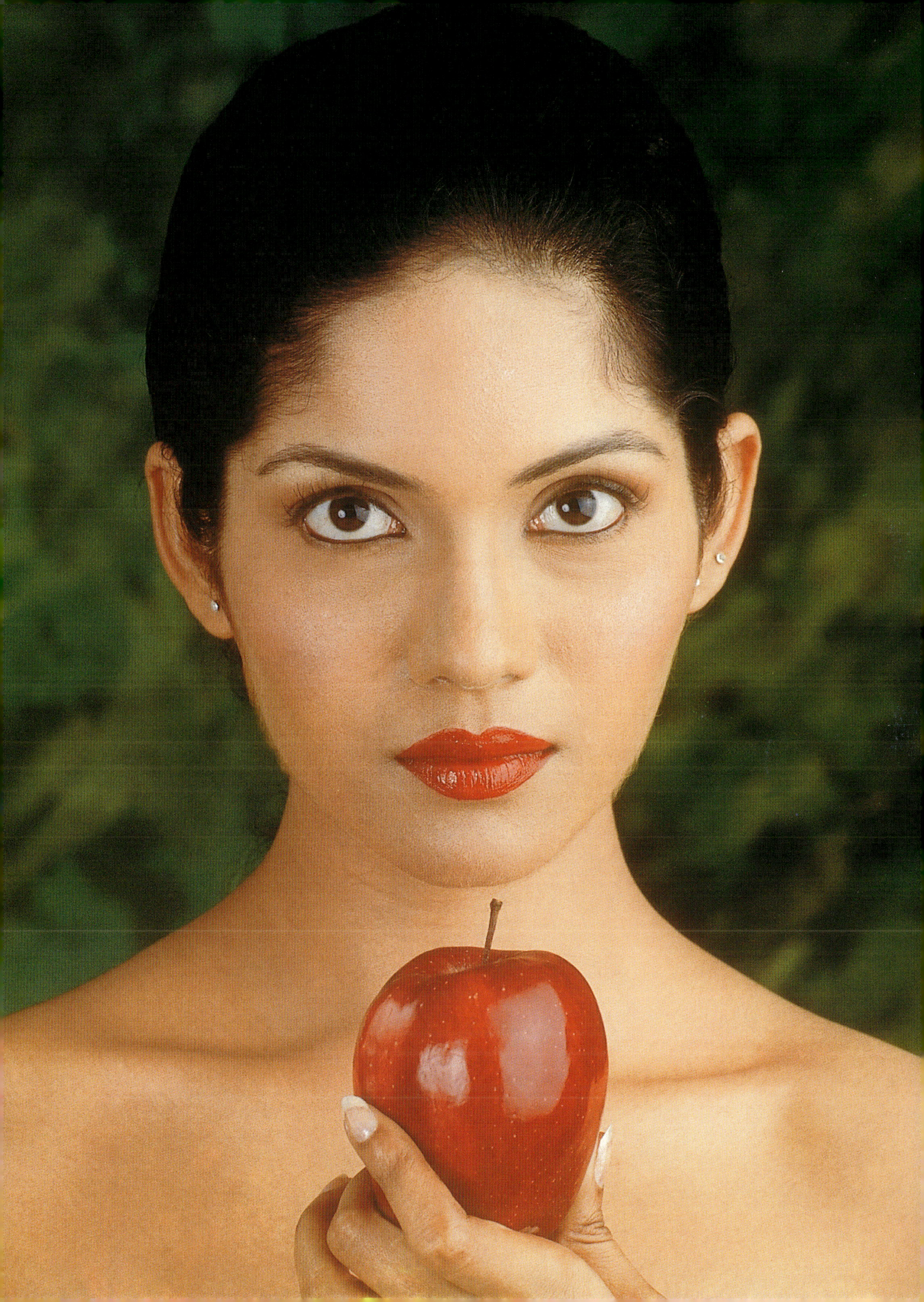

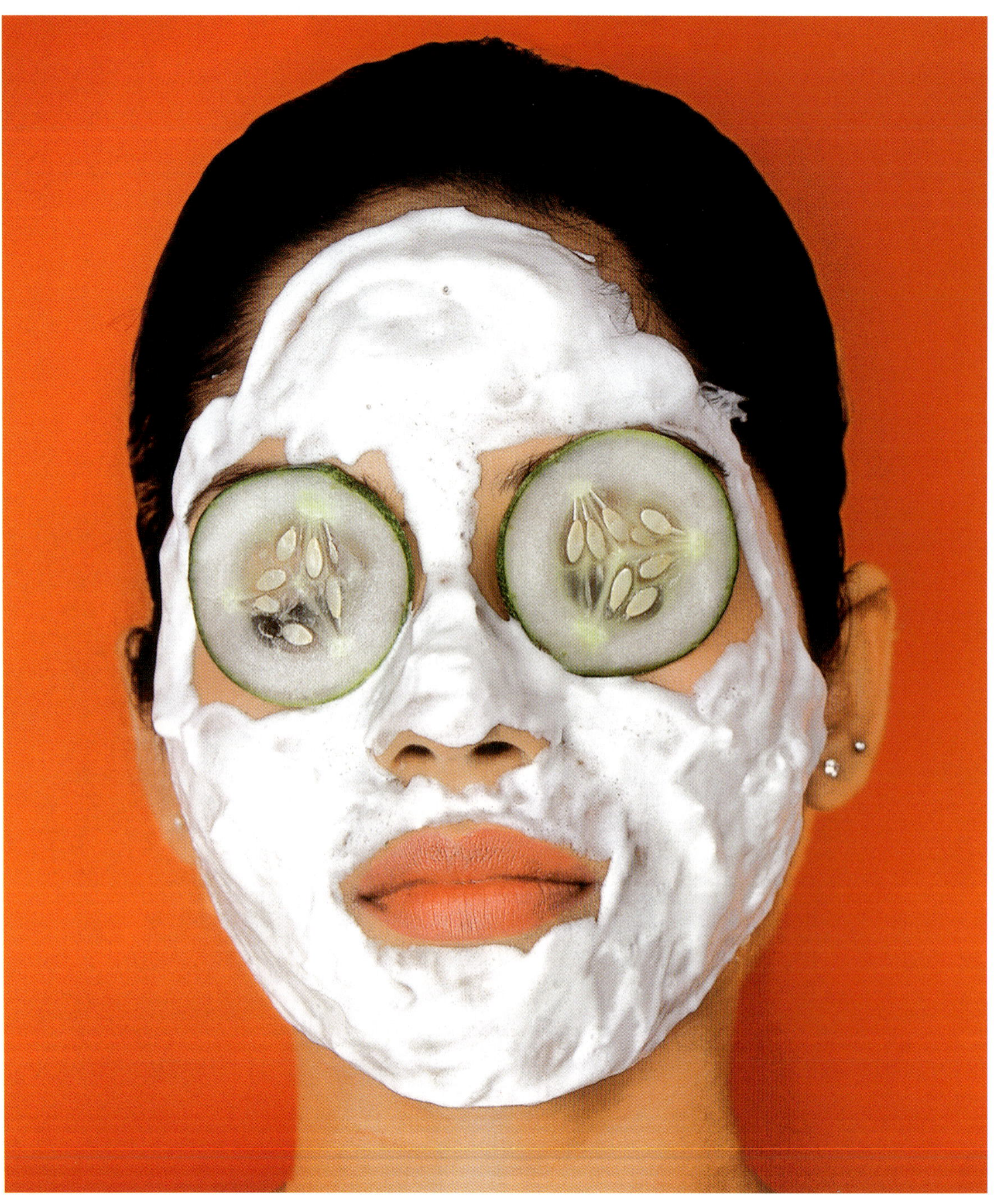

CARROT : Grate 2 carrots and add enough milk to make a thick, non-dripping paste. Spread it evenly all over the face, forehead and the neck. Leave it on for 20 minutes then wash off. This mask rejuvenates the skin.

Another very effective mask can be made with grated carrots and egg yolk. Add beaten egg yolk to the grated carrots and add one teaspoon of almond or olive oil. Mix well in a blender to form a smooth paste. Apply all over the forehead, face and neck. Leave it on for 15 minutes. Use cotton wool dipped in warm milk to wipe it off. Follow with a rinse.

RICE FLOUR : Take a cup of rice powder and to this add enough milk and rosewater to make a thick paste. Apply evenly all over the forehead, face and the neck area. Leave it on for at least 20 minutes. Try and relax and not move any facial muscles when this paste is applied on the face. After 20–30 minutes when it cakes up, splash cold water on your face, rinse and wash off. The skin appears very taut and the wrinkles seem to have "straightened" out or disappeared altogether. Use this treatment regularly, twice or thrice a week for best results.

APRICOT : Wrinkles due to tiredness or tension are quickly removed with this wonderful treatment. Take 2 apricots, after de-seeding them, finely chop and puree along with their skin. Add 2 tablespoons of honey and the juice of one lime along with a little cold milk. Blend all these to form a smooth paste. Apply on the forehead, face and the neck. Leave it on for at least 30 minutes. Now take some lukewarm water in a basin and add to it the juice of one lemon. Wash your face with this water. Your face glows and radiates freshness. The worry and furrow lines are minimized. The apricot nourishes while the lime juice tightens the skin.

EGG AND LIME : Take an egg white and beat it well to form peaks. Now add to it the juice of one lime and blend well. Apply all over the forehead, face and neck. Leave it on for 10 minutes. Wash off with lukewarm water. This tightens the skin instantly.

GREEN GRAPES : Green seedless grapes are also an excellent cure for wrinkles. Roughly crush a few green seedless grapes and apply them on the forehead, face and neck. Rub the grapes in circular motions on all these areas. Leave them on for 20 minutes. Rinse off with water. Regular use controls wrinkles.

POTATO : A potato mask effectively improves the skin texture, lightens wrinkles, makes them fainter, and tightens your skin. Take 2 potatoes, peel and grate them. Apply the grated potatoes all over forehead, face and neck. Leave it on for a few minutes. The feeling of "pinching" and tightening of the skin will be acute. Rinse off with cold water. Cleans and tightens the skin.

Helpful Tips

You can improve your looks at any age. Equipped with useful tips, a careful diet and regular exercise, you can make your face glow with health, beauty, and vitality; without having to resort to camouflage techniques. Face care varies with skin type. Here are some useful tips.

- Dry skin needs hydrating and moisturizing treatment.
- Oily skin needs cleansing and freshening.
- Patchy skin needs smoothening and lightening treatment.
- Change in season requires a change in the skin care routine.
- To keep the skin glowing, drink at least 12–15 glasses of water per day.
- Your diet should be rich in raw vegetables and fresh fruits. These hydrate your skin.
- Protect yourself from the harshness of the sun. This is the main cause of skin discolouration, pigmentation and wrinkles.
- Exercise regularly; even a good walking routine will suffice.
- Exercise facial muscles regularly. Rotate your neck slowly, side to side, and loosen the facial muscles.
- Laugh loudly, it helps to exercise the facial muscles.
- Wash your face several times a day.
- Steam your face once a week to clean up clogged pores. After steaming, rub your face, forehead and neck vigorously to exfoliate the skin.
- Take Vitamin E for shadows and scars. But consult a doctor first.
- Once a fortnight go in for an elaborate cleansing and moisturizing treatment by using any of the fruits and vegetables mentioned. The type and the nature of the treatment depends upon your skin type.
- "Feed" your skin. It requires nourishment too.
- Whenever you apply a lotion or cream or moisturizer, use gentle, swift, featherlike upward strokes. Do not use downward strokes or pull your facial muscles downward, else they will start sagging.
- Whenever you dry your face, always pat it dry. Do not rub, scrub or pull your skin.
- Avoid rapid or excessive weight loss.
- Ensure a good night's sleep. It rests and nourishes your skin.
- A diet rich in Vitamin A prevents a patchy, dry or rough skin. It is also good for people who have acne and pimples.
- Vitamin B prevents spots on the face.
- Strawberries are an instant cure for dry skin. Take a few strawberries, puree them. Add to this half cup milk and a tablespoon of glycerine. Shake well, pour in a jar and store in the refrigerator. Use this whenever the skin appears to be dry and taut. Apply on face, leave on for 10 minutes. Rinse. The skin is as soft like that of a baby.
- Your face is the most expressive, noticeable and also the most delicate part of the body. Normal facial expressions like frowning, raising of the eyebrows, wrinkling of the forehead, all this eventually lead to wrinkles. So make a facial massage as a regular routine to combat wrinkling.
- Use a moisturizer after exfoliation. It helps to reseal the skin and protects it form over drying.
- Prolonged use of alcohol based perfumes and deodorants can cause brown patches and dryness.
- Avoid going out in the direct sun when using a perfume. Spray onto clothes instead of directly on the skin.

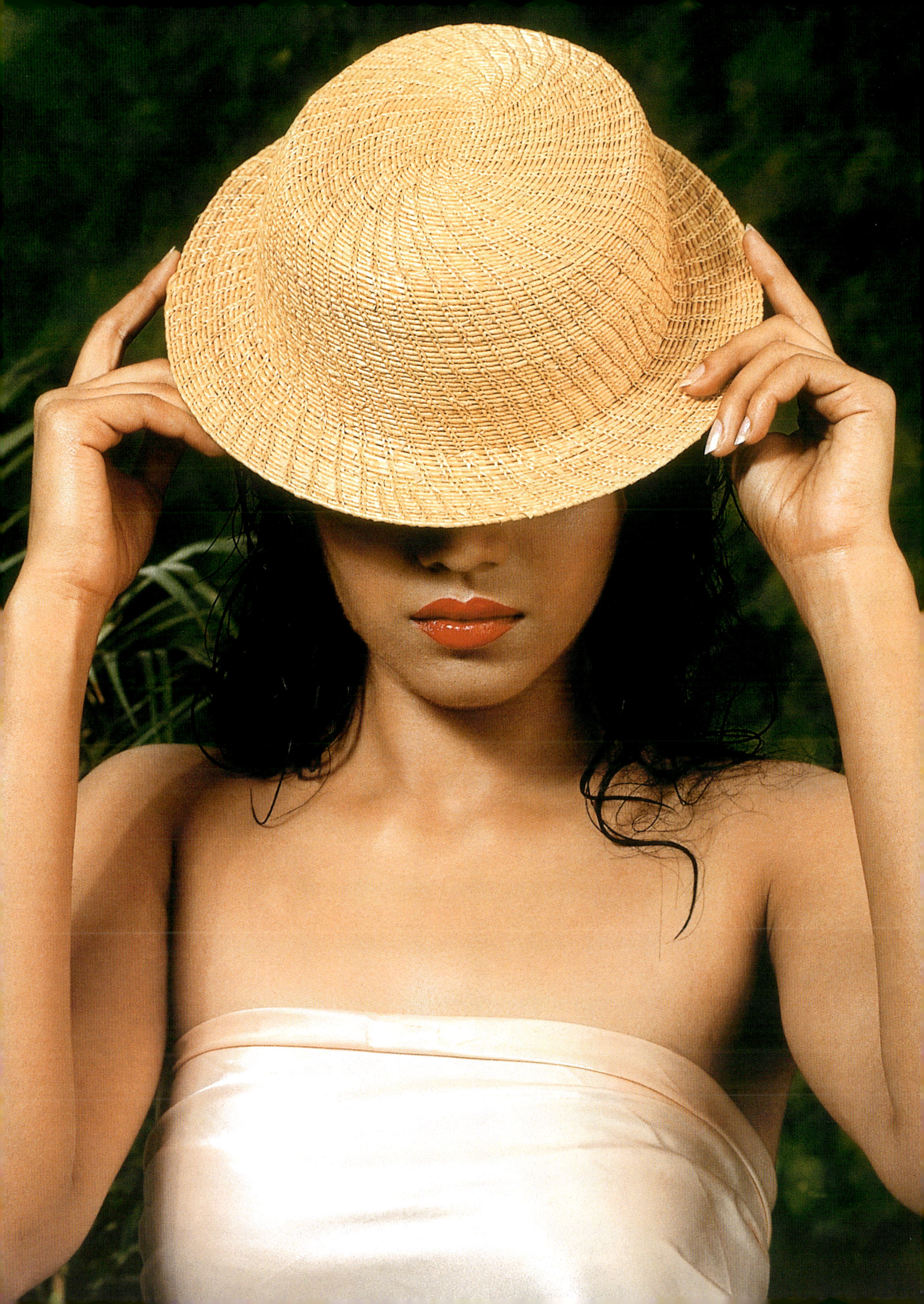

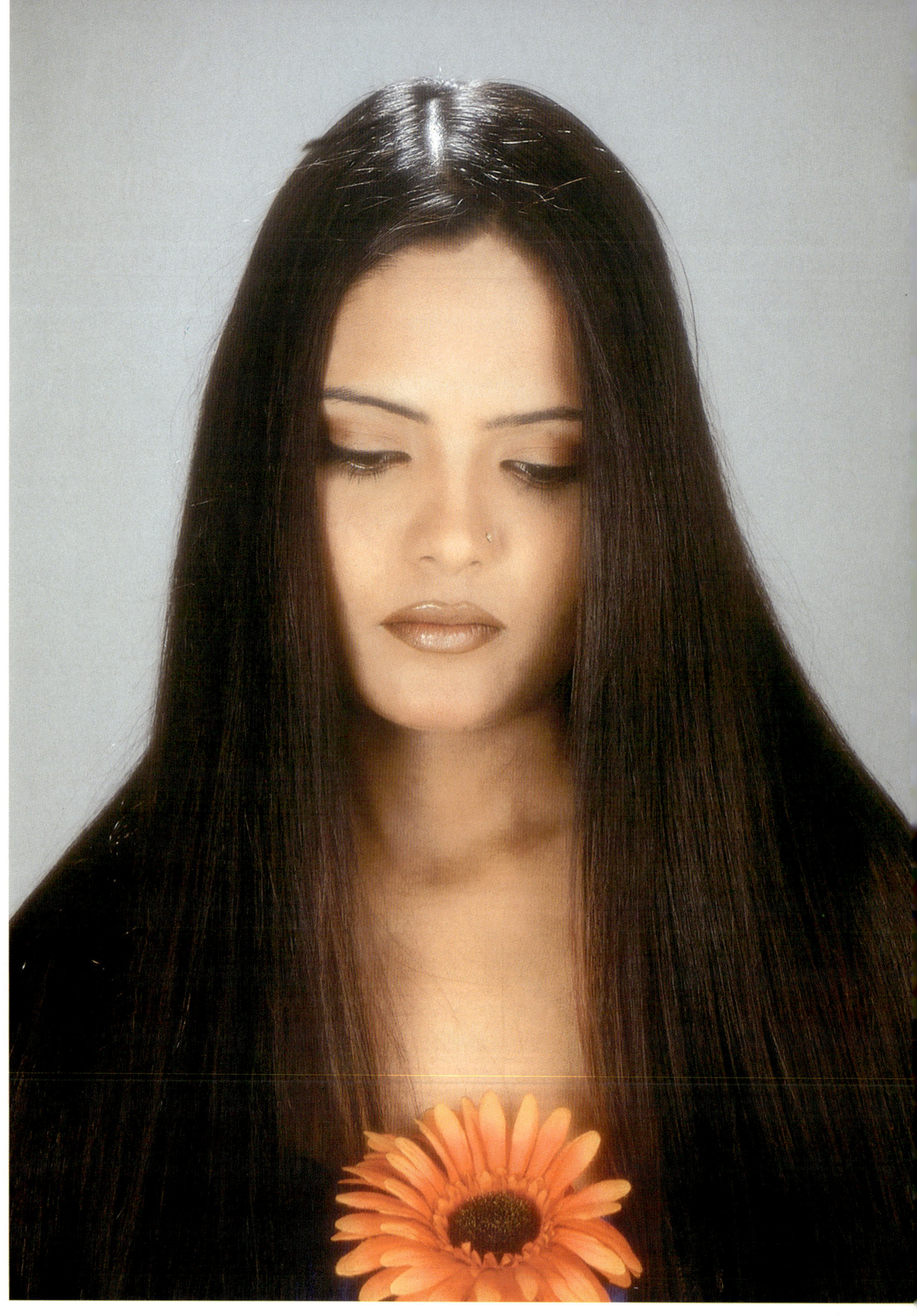

hair
Your Crowning Glory

Long, flowing, lustrous hair has always been associated with women of great beauty. Hair has also been an instrument of fashion, in fact it is often termed as a person's 'crowning glory'. Beautiful, bouncy hair reflects the health of a person; gives the appearance of vibrancy and life. Hair itself is organically dead material, but its follicles are not. The beauty and health of your hair depends upon the health of these follicles. Women spend fortunes on their hair. Well-groomed, luxuriant, lustrous, hair is, quite simply, beautiful and sexy. It can signify youth, health, and vitality.

Hair goes through enormous "tortures" before it is made cosmetically acceptable to most women. Endless hours are spent combing, blow drying, tinting, curling, crimping, straightening, dying and bleaching. In fact, hair is subjected to endless experimentation. Indeed, it has amazing strength and resilience to cope with the vagaries of a woman's mind.

A woman's worst nightmare is loss of hair leading to baldness. Premature greying, rough and brittle hair are some of the numerous problems waiting to be solved. Hair comes in different textures, shades, colours, and is perhaps also a mark of distinction that differentiates between different races.

First, however, we need to know a few basic hair facts. Each hair is made up of an outer layer or cuticle. This is made up of a protein called Keratin, which protects the hair and helps retain moisture. Next is the inner layer where the colouring or pigmentation is produced. This surrounds the innermost layer, the medulla. Hair grows from a follicle on the scalp. Each follicle produces only one strand of hair. An average human head contains between 80,000 to 150,000 strands of hair.

A person's overall health is immediately reflected in the state of her/his hair. A healthy person sports thick, glossy hair. While baldness is usually more genetic in nature, a sudden loss of hair has a lot to do with external health factors. For women it could well be due to a reduced level of the hormone estrogen during pregnancy, hair loss due to anxiety and tension, hormonal imbalances, pollution, sudden weight loss, as also a badly mismanaged diet schedule.

The shape of the hair follicle determines your type of hair. Flat, oval shaped follicles promote curly hair, while perfectly round follicles promote straight hair. Hair colour is usually inherited and it complements the shade of the skin. Then, we have hair that is naturally dry or oily, fine or coarse, shiny or dull. There is a great variety.

Some of the most common problems are dandruff, split ends, thinning or falling hair, premature greying, dull and rough hair. Many, if not all of these problems can be tackled at home with natural products made from commonly available fruits, vegetables and herbs.

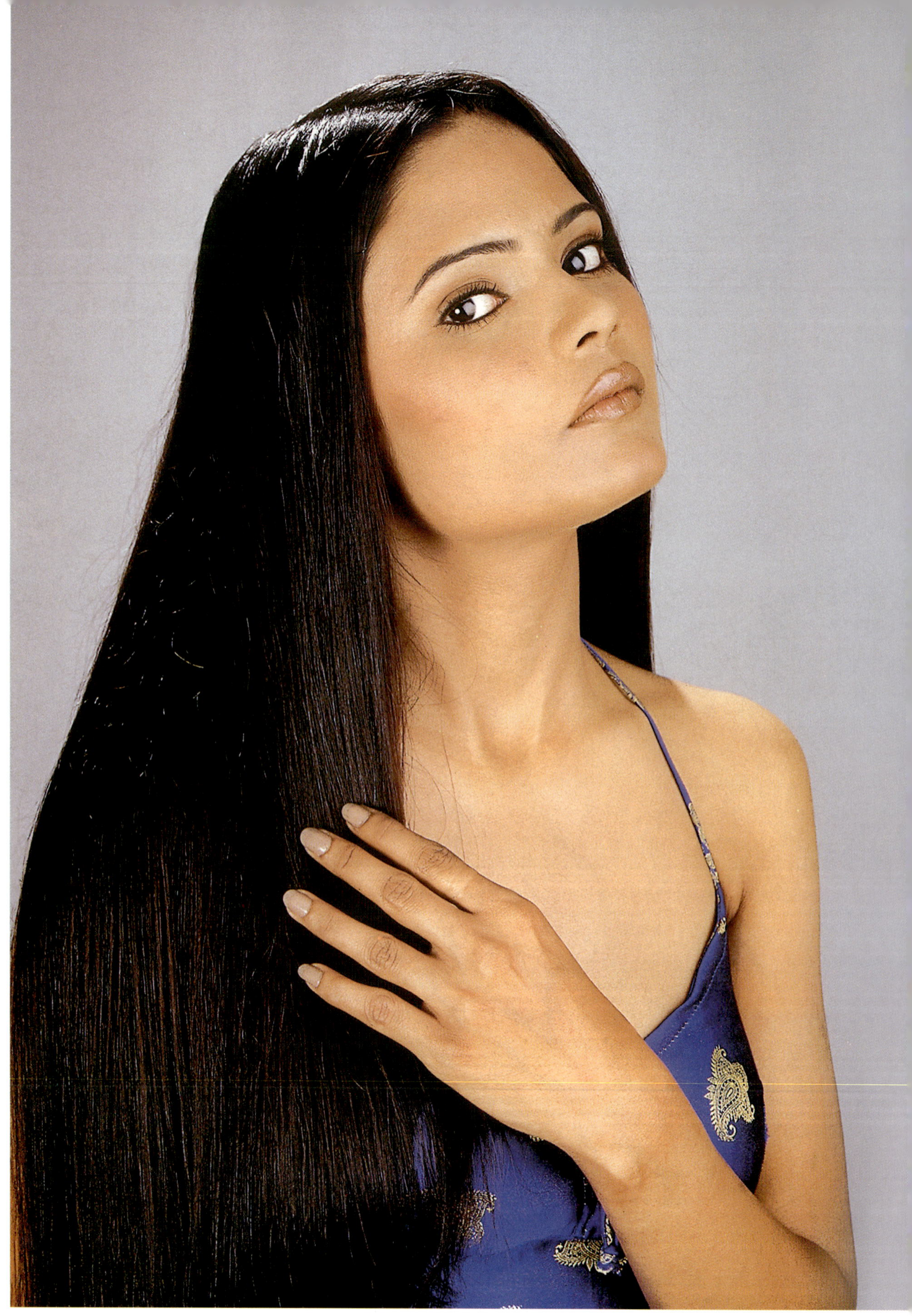

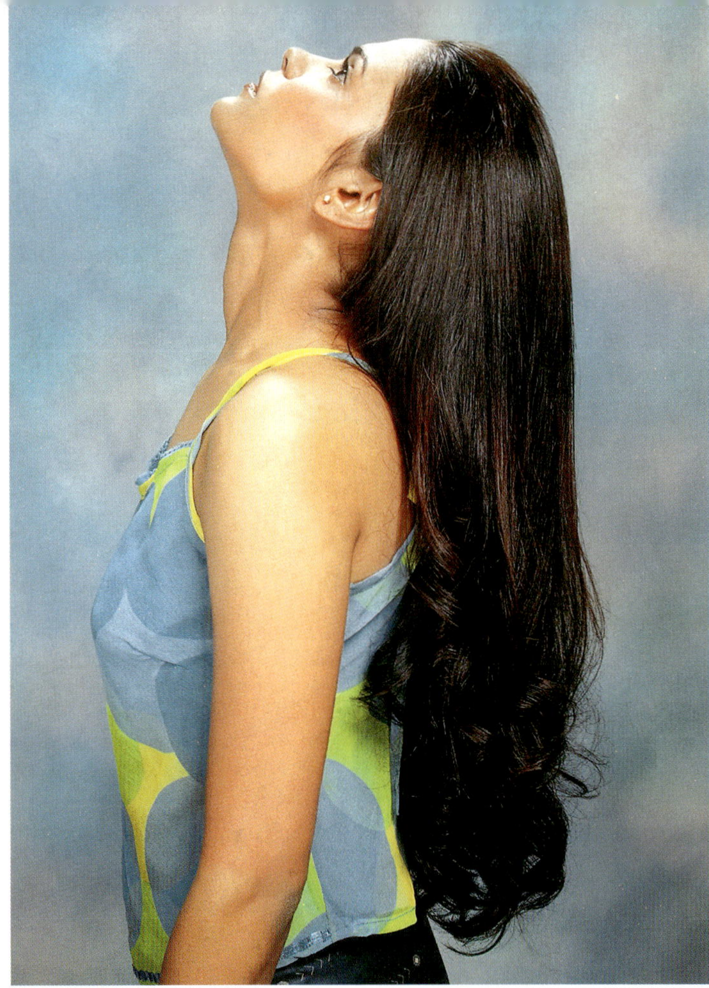

Dandruff

This is the most common complaint, and all of us suffer from this at some time or the other. There are a lot of misconceptions associated with dandruff. People who have this problem rush out and buy up the latest shampoos and conditioners.

There is also a misconception that dandruff is caused by dry scalp. In fact, it is due to an oily scalp. Wrong dietary habits like excessive consumption of cheese and chocolates also cause oil to accumulate on the scalp and cause dandruff. Worry and tension increase the flow of oil in the scalp, make you prone to dandruff. These white flakes can be a nightmare. Dandruff further tends to weaken the scalp, and the flakes falling on your face, neck and shoulders can affect your skin too.

WARM OIL TREATMENT : Warm 4-5 tablespoons full of wheat germ oil, olive oil or coconut oil. Massage well into the scalp. Wrap a warm towel around your head. Leave it on for 30 minutes. Rinse your hair thoroughly with water, to which lemon juice has been added. Massage well as you rinse. This is the most commonly known cure for dandruff.

CHICKPEA FLOUR (BESAN) AND CURD : Take half a cup of chickpea flour. Add to this a little curd and enough water to make a thick paste. Apply on the scalp and individual strands of hair. Leave it on for for 30 minutes. Rinse vigorously with warm water.

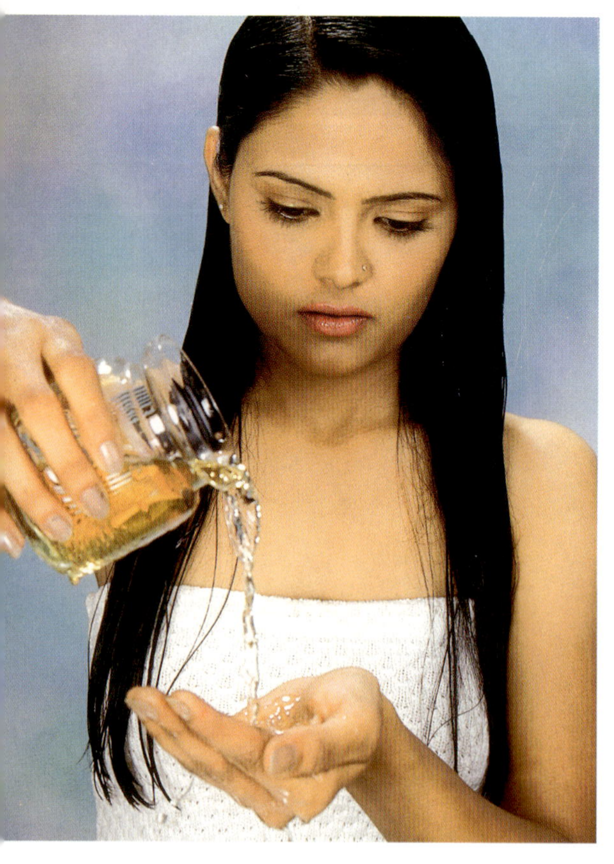

ROSEMARY AND OIL TREATMENT : Take half a cup of coconut or olive oil. Add a few drops of rosemary oil, (alternatively, crush some fresh, or even dry rosemary leaves, boil them in the oil. Let it cool, then strain the oil by squeezing the leaves.) Apply all over the scalp. Leave it on all night after wrapping up your head with a towel. In the morning, rinse your hair with a mixture of warm water and lemon juice.

FENUGREEK (METHI) SEEDS AND OIL : Crush a tablespoon of fenugreek seeds in about 5 tablespoons of warm coconut or olive oil. It would be better to boil them in the oil. Cool the mixture and apply generously all over the scalp. Leave it it on for two hours. Rinse and wash off.

SOAP NUT (REETHA) : This is ideal for removing dandruff. Soak half cup soap nut overnight in one cup of warm water. Extract the juice from the soap nut by rubbing them vigorously. Strain. Apply directly on the scalp. Leave this on for 15 minutes. Rinse and wash your hair with tepid water. Shut your eyes tightly while rinsing as it hurts the eyes. Ensure that no residue is left behind.

ONION : Grind raw onions to a fine paste. Rub this paste into your scalp. Leave it on for an hour. Wash thoroughly. Rub in some lemon juice into your scalp and hair to rid your self of the onion smell.

BLACK PEPPER : Take 10 grams of black pepper powder. Add to it the juice of a fresh lime, along with a quarter cup of milk. Rub this mixture thoroughly into your scalp. Leave it on for an hour and wash it out thoroughly with water.

Dry Lifeless Hair

This hair looks like unwashed straw. It grows thicker nearer the scalp and thins out towards the ends, thus causing split ends. Atmospheric pollution too tends to have a drying effect on the hair. Such hair needs extra care.

WARM OIL MASSAGE : The is nothing as nourishing as a warm oil massage. Take half a cup of coconut oil. Crush 4 almonds and add to oil. Steam this mixture by placing it inside a pan. Apply while still warm, deep into the scalp and into the roots of your hair. Cover your head with a towel and leave it on for half an hour. Shampoo your hair.

BANANA NOURISHING PACK : Mash two ripe bananas. Add half cup beaten curd. Apply this paste all over your scalp and coat the ends of the hair with it. Pile up your

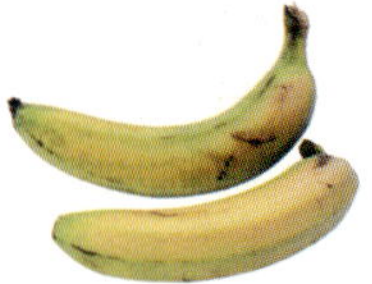

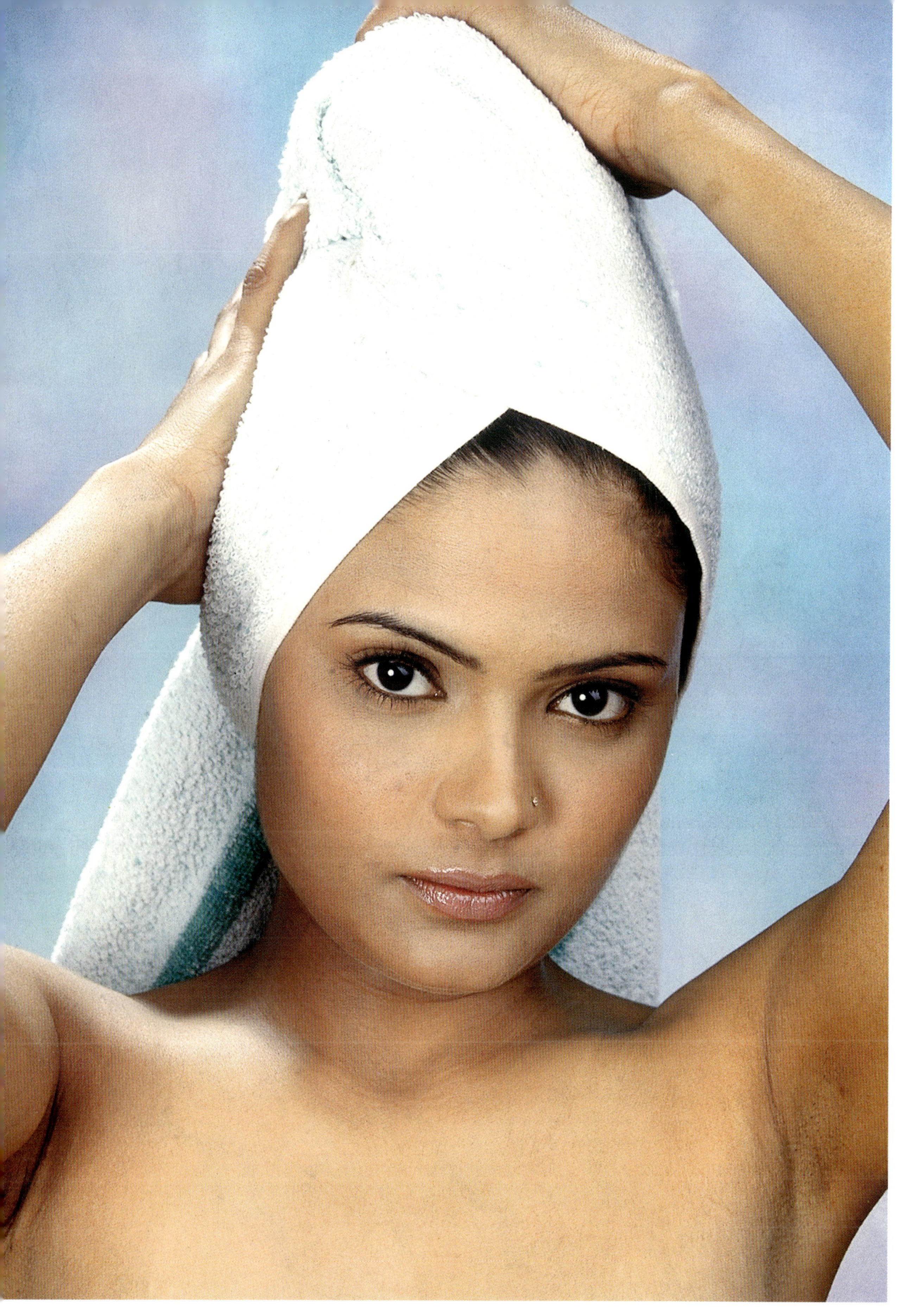

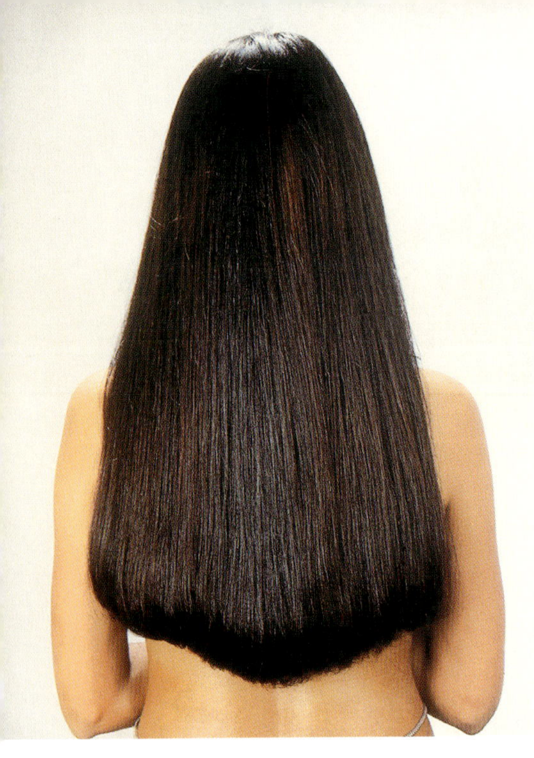

hair high over your head. Leave it on for 15 minutes and then shampoo as usual. You will immediately notice a dramatic change in the texture of your hair.

EGG TONIC : Beat up an egg in a cup of milk. Squeeze in the juice of one lemon. Add to this a teaspoon of coconut oil or olie oil Massage well into your hair. Cover with moist, warm towel. Leave it on for an hour. Rinse it thoroughly. The final rinse should be with lime juice and warm water. A good alternative would be to add yogurt instead of the milk.

Split Ends

To treat split ends, first trim off the ends of your hair to an even length. Use all the nourishing applications described in the earlier chapter for your hair. Avoid back-combing or use of spiky rollers. You could also use these other nourishing tonic applications for your hair.

PAPAYA PACK : A unique, simple and easy remedy to bring your hair back to life. Take half of a ripe medium sized papaya. Slice after skinning and deseeding it. Put it in a blender and blend it to a pulp. Add half cup of yogurt and apply lavishly to your scalp. Part your hair at regular intervals and apply to hair strands and hair ends. Leave it on for 30 minutes. Rinse hair thoroughly with warm water.

CREAM TONIC : After you shampoo your hair, use the following tonic: take half cup milk; add to this a tablespoon of cream. Beat it up. Apply on scalp, hair strands and hair ends. Leave it on for 15 minutes. Rinse and wash well with water.

HONEY : Take half a cup of curd. Add to this a table spoon full of honey. Mix well. Apply on scalp and hair strands and hair ends. After 20 minutes wash with water. See a remarkable change in the sheen and smoothness of your hair.

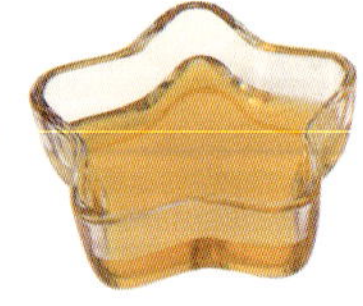

BLACK LENTIL PACK : Take half a cup of black dal (lentil). Add one table spoon of fenugreek (methi) seeds. Dry grind to a coarse powder. Add half a cup of curd. Mix well. Apply generously all over the scalp. Leave it on for 2 hours. Wash your hair with water using a mild shampoo.

Any of these treatments should be a regular part of the attention that your hair deserves from you. The results? Seeing is believing.

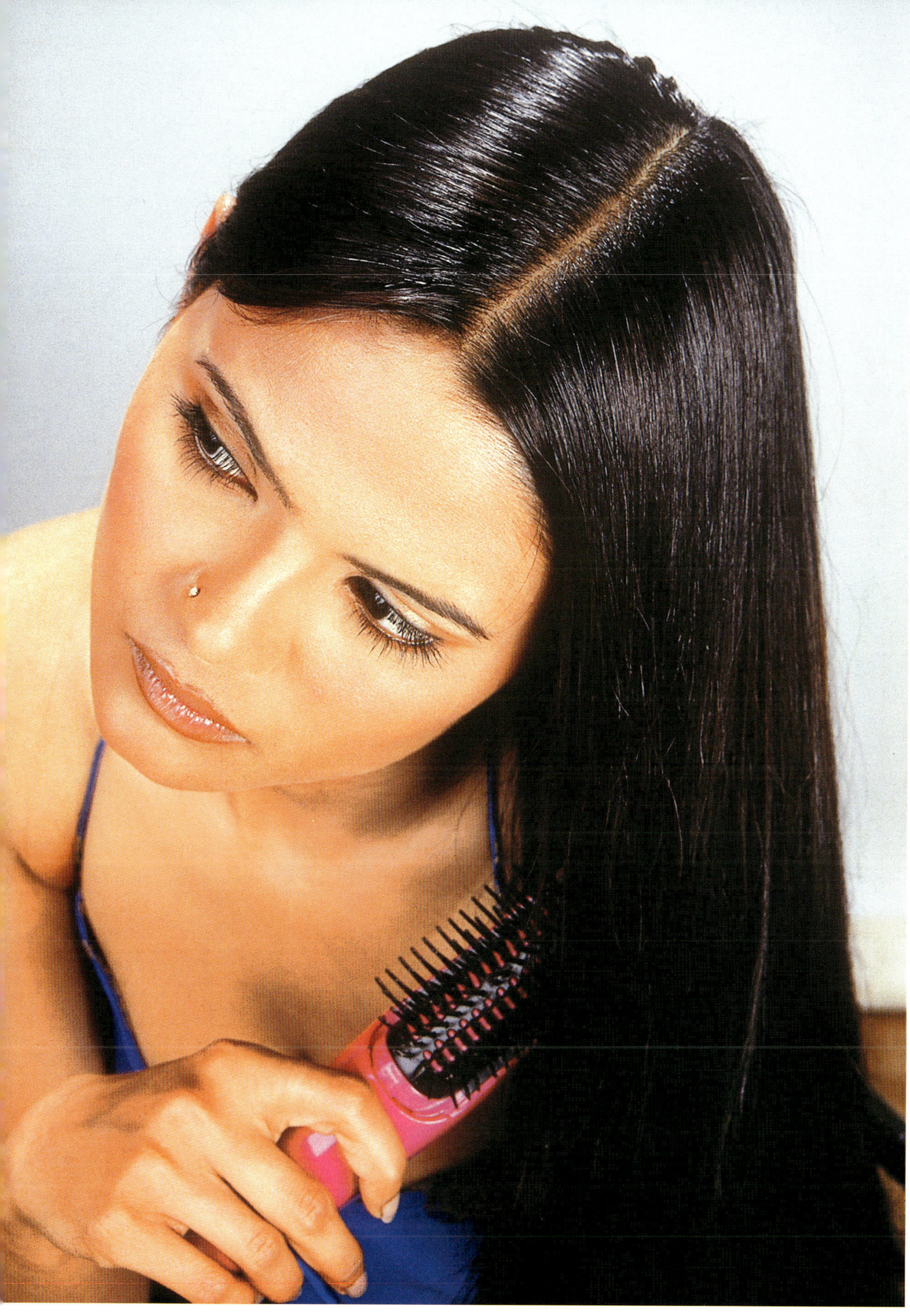

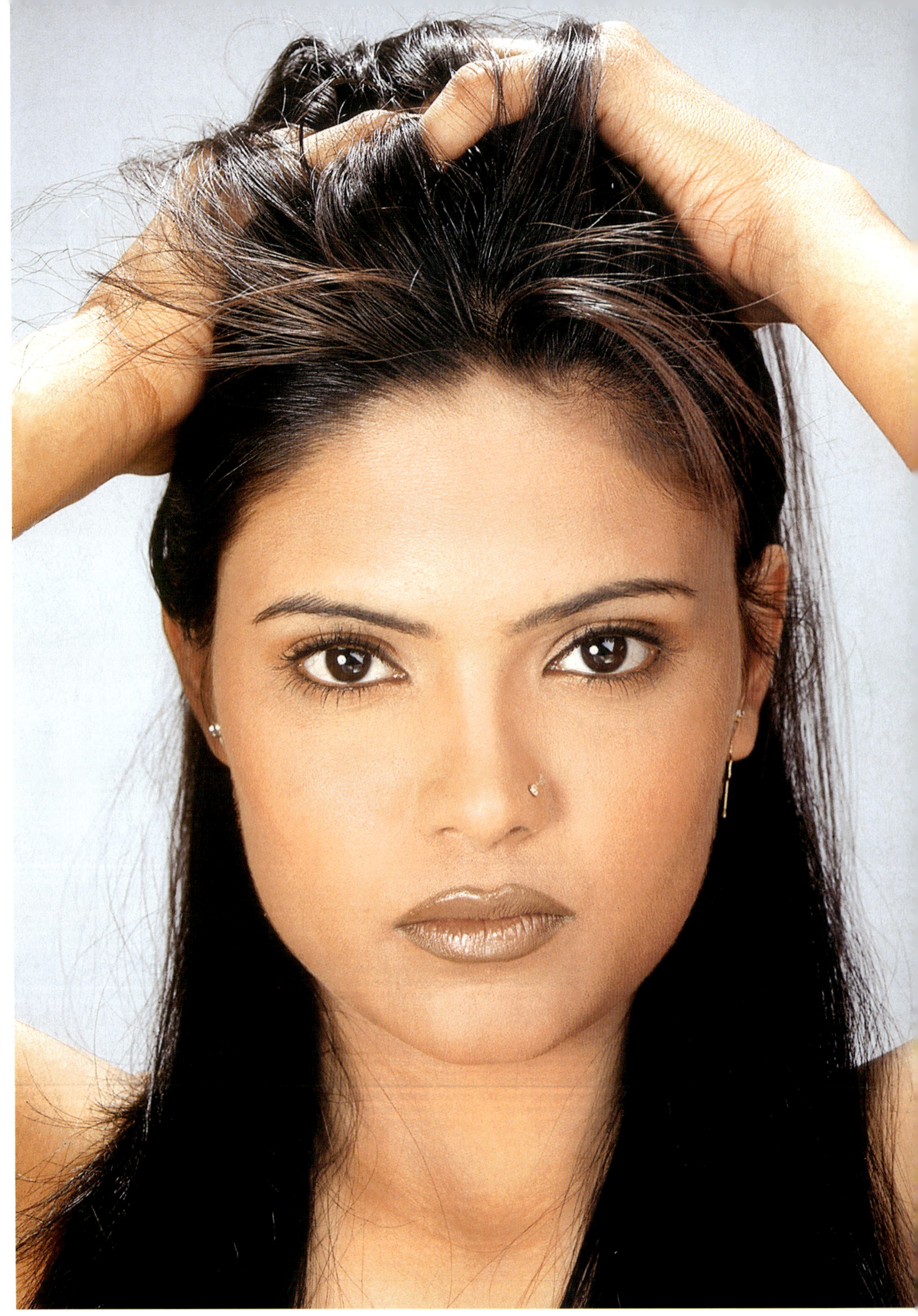

Greying Hair

The pigment Melanin controls the colouring of your hair. With advancing age, the quantity of pigment produced decreases, and your hair starts greying. Heredity too plays a major role in greying of hair. Pollution in the atmosphere and high chlorine content in water play havoc with your hair and cause premature greying. Natural treatment can arrest and delay this process. The watchword? Patience and continuity of treatment.

SAGE AND TEA APPLICATION : Put 2 tablespoons tea leaves and a handful of sage in a pan. Add half litre of water. Let it boil for 5 minutes. Cool sufficiently, strain the concoction and apply it to the roots of the hair. A very effective hair darkener.

HENNA : The universal favourite since the beginning of time. Used for colouring and covering grey hair. Acts as a tonic too, but has a drying effect; therefore best used along with a mixture of amla powder, boiled tea leaves in water and a little mustard oil. Apply this paste on your hair and leave it on for 2 hours. Wash off with water.

ONION PASTE : Few are aware of the magical properties of onion for your hair. Regular use of onion paste restores the original colour to your hair. Again, be patient and regular.

BLACK PEPPER AND CURD PACK : Take half cup curd. Add to this one tablespoon of ground black pepper and the juice of one lemon. Apply this paste on your hair. Regular use helps in darkening your hair and the restoration of pigmentation.

WALNUT APPLICATION : Crush the fruit of the walnut and power the outer shell. Boil in water. Strain and keep aside till it cools. Use generously and massage deep into your scalp. Leave it on for 20 minutes, then rinse with water. Helps in the retention of pigmentation of your hair.

FENUGREEK (METHI) APPLICATION : Powder fenugreek seeds or chop fenugreek leaves very fine and boil in mustard oil. Cool, strain and then apply on your hair. Controls pigmentation loss.

AMLA, SHIKAKAI APPLICATION : Take 5 tablespoons of amla powder; 5 tablespoons of shikakai power and 2 tablespoons of tea leaves. Put them on to boil. Pour the entire contents into an iron wok (karhai). Leave it overnight. The herbs absorb the iron from the wok and the mixture turns a deep black. Apply this thick paste all over your scalp, ensure that the strands and hair ends are also coated. Leave on for 30 minutes. Rinse and wash off with water.

BITTER GOURD (KARELA) APPLICATION : Chop the bitter gourd along with the skin into thick round pieces. Soak in a bowl containing 1 cup coconut oil. Leave it for 4 days. Boil, cool and strain after squeezing the bitter gourd juice into the oil. Use this oil regularly. Helps in darkening the hair and restoration of pigmentation.

Oily Hair

This type of hair is very fine in texture. It is easily affected by atmospheric pollution and needs to be shampooed and washed more often. If you have oily hair, then try and keep it covered when going out in the sun. Diet too is important. Avoid fried foods and dairy products. Increase your intake of fresh fruits, green and leafy vegetables and salads. Drink plenty of water.

LIME AND VINEGAR RINSE : Take a cup of warm water and add three tablespoons of vinegar along with the juice of one lemon. Gently massage this mixture into your hair and scalp. Leave it on for 30 minutes. Wash and rinse with water.

ALMOND OIL AND WATER APPLICATION : Take half cup water, add to this a teaspoonful of almond oil. Massage this into your hair half an hour prior to your bath. Shampoo and rinse off. Note, the massage is with oil and water emulsion. Do not use only the oil.

BAKING SODA RINSE : The hair accumulates dirt very quickly. In addition, there is a build up of shampoo and conditioner . It alters the alkaline (pH) levels, making the hair oily and limp. Here is a quick rejuvenation application. Take a tablespoon of baking soda, add to it 4 tablespoons of cider vinegar. Rub this into your scalp, leave it on for 5-7 minutes and shampoo your hair. It comes out squeaky clean, vivacious and buoyant.

COLOGNE RUB : Mix equal parts of any cologne and water. Use cotton wool to rub this mixture into fine partings of the hair. This lifts grease of the roots. Wash hair as usual.

APPLE AND VINEGAR RINSE : Grate one apple. Add to it half cup vinegar. Apply generously all over scalp and length of hair. Leave it on for 20 minutes, wash off, rinse thoroughly.

TEA RINSE: Make a tea rinse by boiling tea leaves in water. Squeeze in juice of one lime. Strain and keep aside. After a shampoo use this rinse. Leave it on for 20 minutes, wash off, rinse thoroughly.

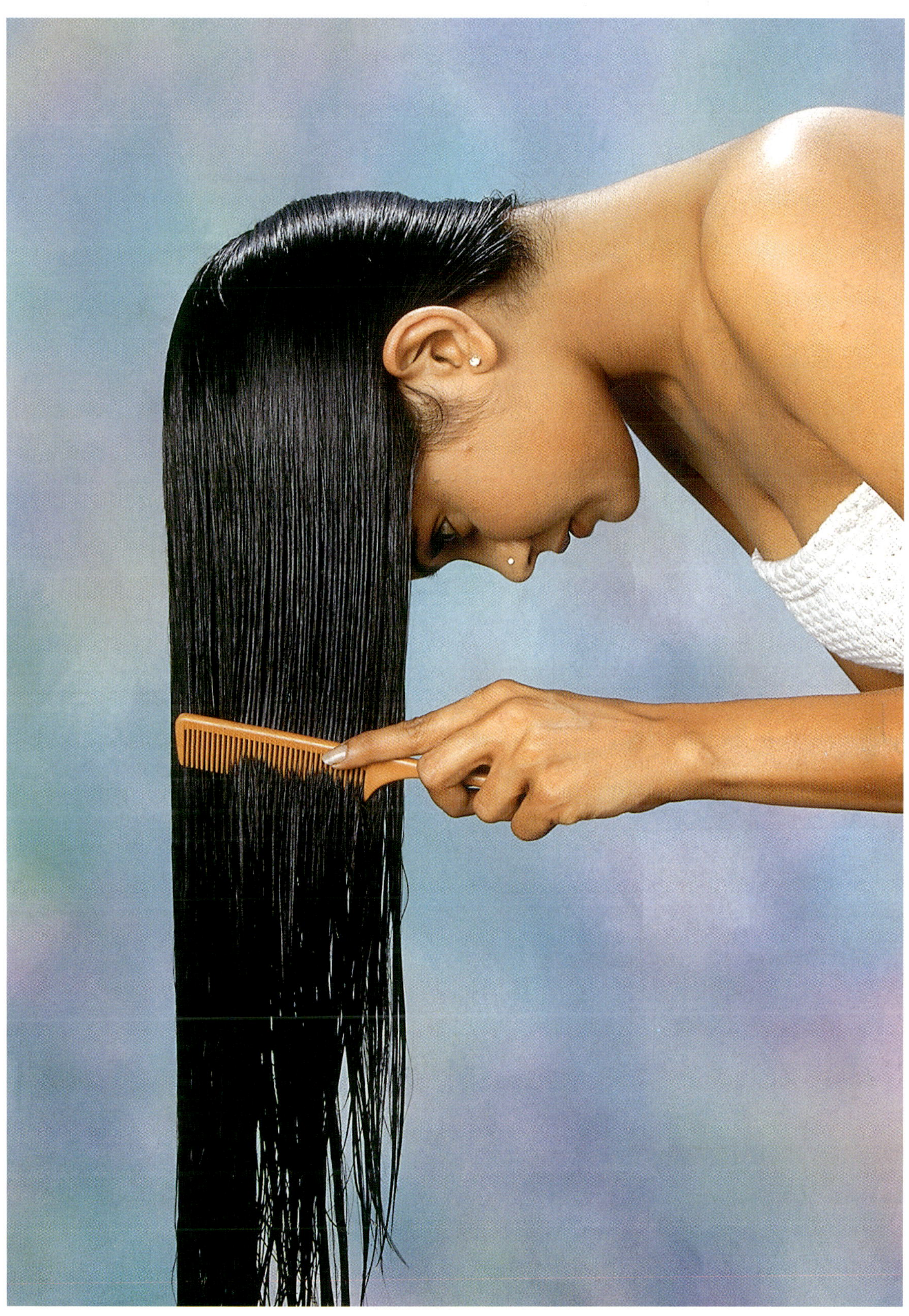

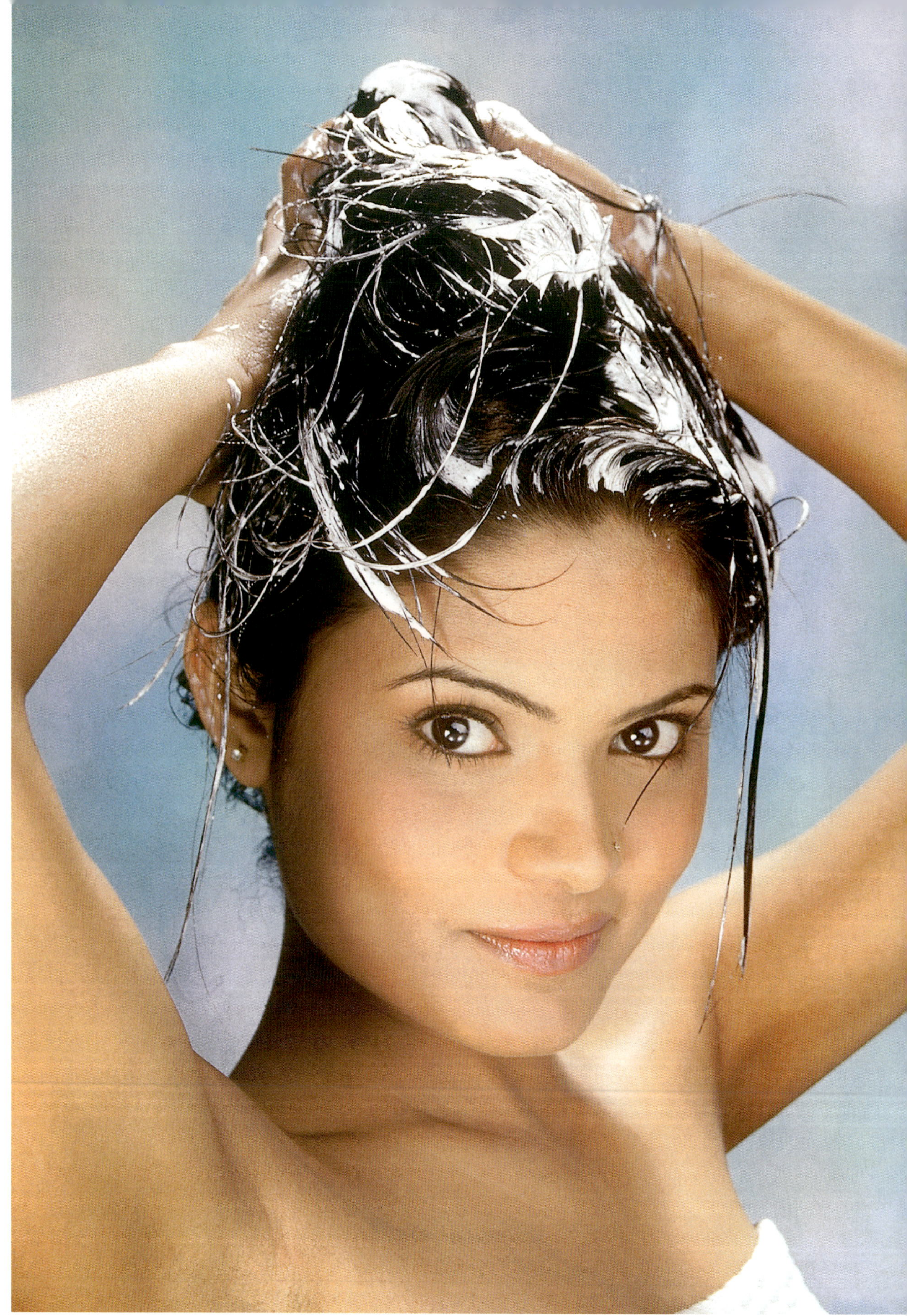

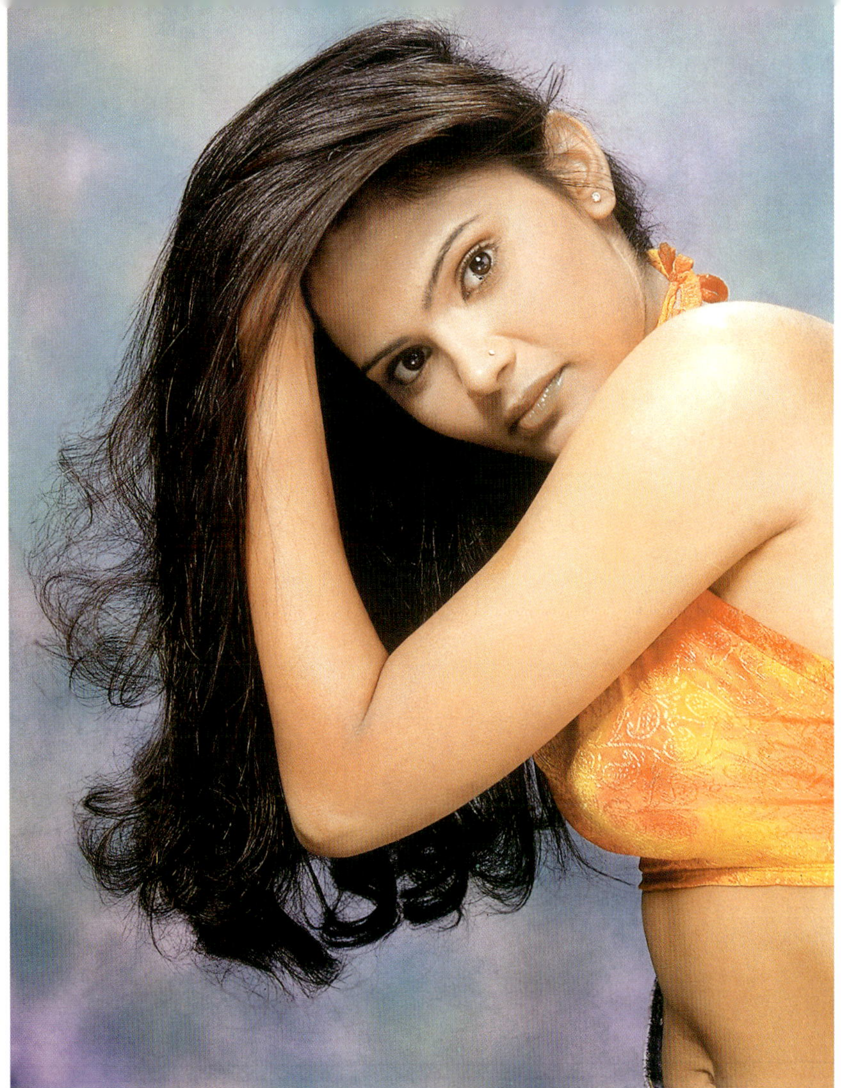

Homemade Hair Conditioners

Fruits, vegetables and even nourishing food are miraculous hair conditioners if used in the right way.

AVOCADO : Chop and put fruit in blender. Mix 2 egg yolks in this pulp. Massage well into hair. Rinse with a mixture of lime juice and vinegar.

MAYONNAISE : Food for hair! Heat half cup of mayonnaise. Apply to dry, unwashed hair. Leave it on for half an hour. Rinse, then shampoo. Gives super results.

SAFFRON : Boil saffron strands in water. Cool it. Add to it the juice of one lime and one tablespoon of honey. Rub into scalp and hair strands. Leave it on for 15 minutes. Rinse thoroughly with water. Your hair acquires a golden sheen.

Helpful Tips

Some people are genetically prone to grey hair, thinning hair or balding. However, the health of your hair depends largely on your blood circulation and nutrition. Without adequate protein inputs in our body, hair stops growing. Its colour changes and it becomes brittle and lifeless. Thus, ensure that you have protein with foods.

Sometimes low haemoglobin results in hair loss. This is due to iron deficiency, which can be overcome by eating bananas, apples and other iron enriched foods.

Avoid eating refined foods like chocolates, burgers, pizzas and pastries. Yeast tablets help hair growth, so does Vitamin E. Other foods that promote hair growth are grains, beans, lentils, green leafy vegetables particularly fenugreek, carrot juice, beetroot juice, fish and fruits like avocado, apple and banana. Here are a few tips for your crowning glory.

* A regular hair care regime should be followed.
* Tie a scarf if you are going out in the hot sun. A hundred strokes at night as granny advised should not be forgotten. Brush firmly, but not harshly, by putting your head forward and throwing your hair in front. Brush neck downwards and outwards.
* A warm oil massage regularly is a must.
* Be careful when using a conditioner, avoid using it on the scalp, only on the hair strands.
* Do not apply the shampoo directly onto the hair. Take a little water in the palm of your hand and mix the shampoo first before applying on the hair.
* After shampooing your hair, it is always better to rinse the hair too.
* Occasionally rinse your hair with some of the rinses mentioned above.
* Choose the right kind of brush for your hair. Flat brushes are best for normal use. Use round and vented brushes for blow drying, while a cushioned brush body is best because it moulds itself to your contours.
* Always ensure that you follow a regular cleaning and nourishing routine.
* So it is about going back to the basics. It is about healthy hair, and feeling good with a little help from nature.

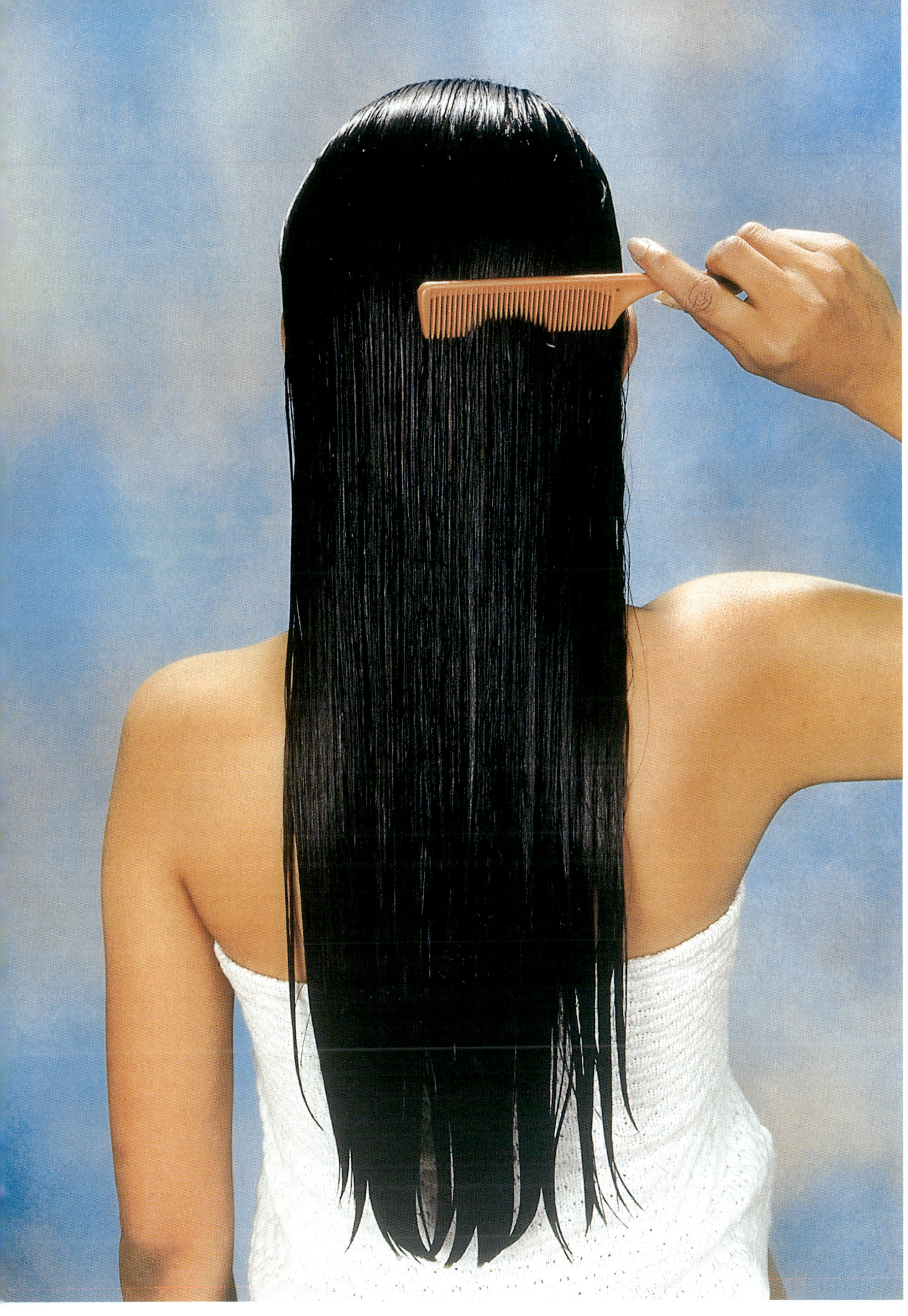

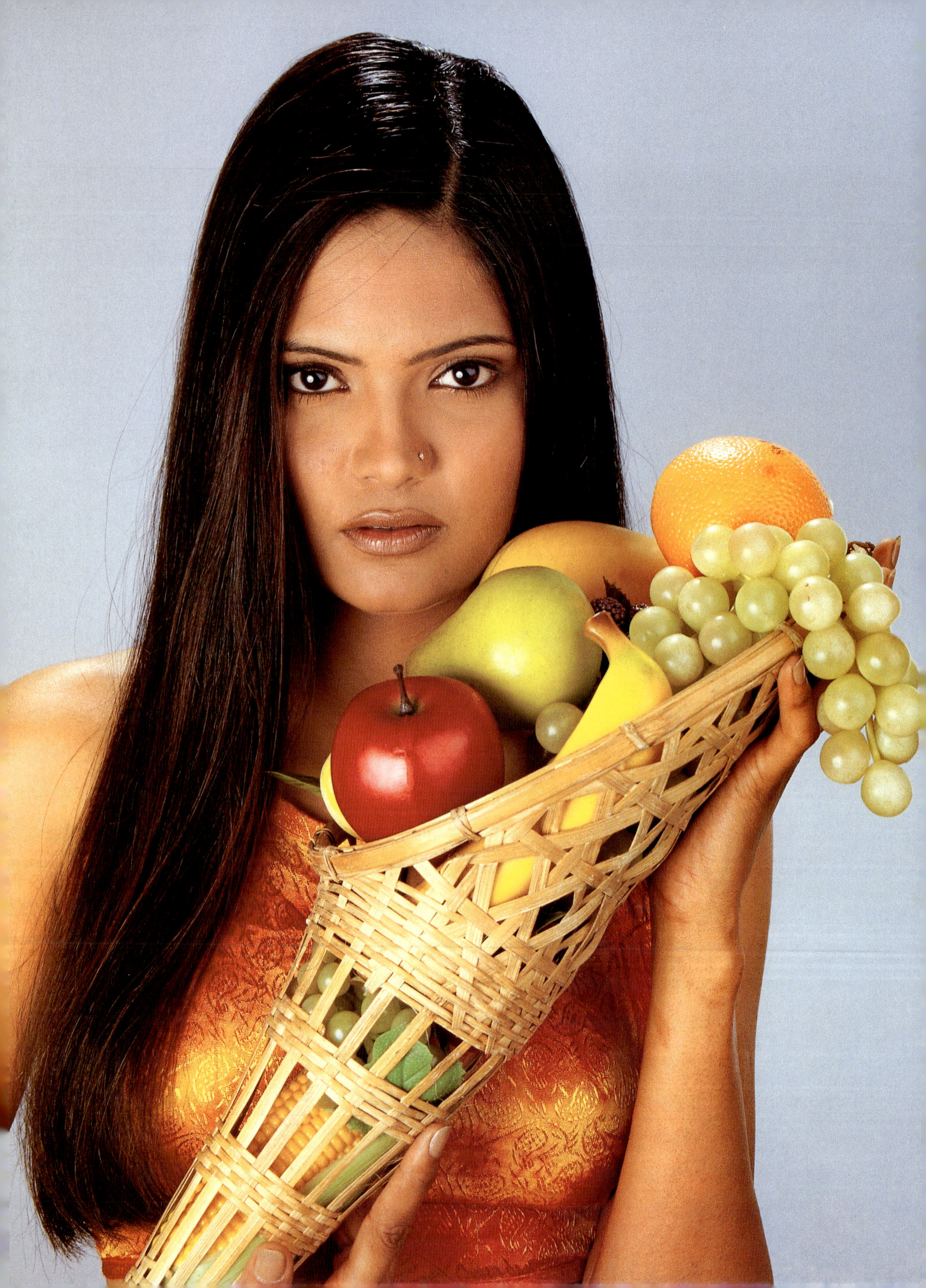

Eat and Grow Beautiful

Looking beautiful and retaining one's beauty should not make you an obsessive slave to beauty cures. While the right use of make-up and beauty care products can undoubtedly enhance your beauty, you can be truly beautiful only if you are healthy. So, eat the right food and grow beautiful. Once you gain knowledge about the right kinds of foods for good health, you can start eating a well-regulated diet, and the results will only be too evident. Your face will glow with health and vitality, your hair will bounce and shine, and your body will be taut and trim. It makes a lot of sense to care not only about the food you eat, but also in the manner in which you do so. A few tips on practical knowledge about food and eating habits would certainly go a long way into developing a healthy regime, which will stand you in good stead.

Undoubtedly, beauty is also a state of the mind. In order to look good, you ought to "feel good" too. True beauty comes from within; from a feeling of well-being. It is not the way you dress, or do your make-up, nor your sense of style or get up, but it is the person within you that looks radiant and beautiful.

Good looks have a lot more to do with food than is commonly realised. The key to vitality, health and beauty is in eating right.

Women in general, and working women in particular, ignore their basic food requirements, leading to malnourishment and other deficiencies. Today, in any urban environment, as much as 75% of young working women are anaemic. This also results in period cramps, heavy bleeding, abdominal bloating and irritability. All this takes a heavy toll on your body and in the way you look. Coupled with this is the fact that many urban women are prone to emotional dieting fads, which messes up the delicate balance within the body, and deprive themselves of essentials like iron, calcium, proteins and minerals. Eventually, this affects the hair, skin, and teeth, and gives the appearance of premature ageing. Bulimia and Anorexia are also growing as women look to magazines and glossy advertisements and try to be like the thin emasculated models that promote the business of beauty.

Excess of carbohydrates for instance, can take a toll on the hair, skin and the eyes. On the flip side, the addition of vitamins and other nutrients to food can make a difference in the quality of your skin, your hair, and remove headaches and irritability and other day-to-day ailments. Did you know that sluggishness and lack of energy could be overcome with a changed and improved diet plan?

All this does not imply that you need to be fastidious or obsessive about your food. It only means that you need to have basic nutritional awareness about your food. You can thus select the right kinds of foods best suited to the needs of your body. Its your daily food intake that is important. So, do spare a thought for food. Make sure that you get enough nutrients and have a balanced diet. This is the key to good health and beauty. Modern day eating habits, convenient cooking and fast food culture robs us of essentials like vitamin B complex, as found in milk, liver, fish and wheat germ. We tend to cultivate wrong eating habits. Let me just tell you very briefly about some nutrients that are absolutely essential for a sound and healthy body.

SKIN: Your skin needs Vitamin B2. This is present in fresh vegetables, milk, whole wheat bread. It also needs Vitamin C to vitalise and purify the blood-stream. The easy way out? Eat at least one orange a day. Simple!

TEETH AND BONES : These need calcium and Vitamin D. So take plenty of milk and fish. Avoid too much of starch and sugar.

HAIR : Hair is made from a protein-based substance called keratin. Thus, a healthy mane of hair needs plenty of protein and vitamin B. A high protein diet should include fish, cheese and eggs.

NAILS : To avoid chipping, cracking and discolouring of nails, ensure that you have a diet rich in proteins and minerals and iodine.

EYES : The most essential requirement for healthy eyes is Vitamin A. Carrots and cabbage and other leafy vegetables are a good source, as are butter, eggs and fish.

Over the years, our eating habits have deteriorated. Coupled with the fact that pesticides are being used in grains, fruits and vegetables, eventually they rob you of essential "natural" nutrients. Today's working women seek a quick and easy way out. Thus, many people go in for processed foods, which may be the primary cause of poor nutrition. There is really no substitute for nature. We have seen it time and again. Natural produce, fruits, vegetables and food grains are best when grown in its natural process without any artificial ingredients. An increasingly large number of people are depriving themselves of essential nutrients. True, the modern, stressful lifestyle may be a cause, but lack of interest and ignorance about the basic nutritional values is definitely the other cause.

In today's lifestyle, busy people with little time for shopping for food and even lesser time for cooking it, do not realise the harmful effects of only relying on processed foods. Besides, the marketing hype and fashion cults often change, dictate and shape people's food habits. Be wary of such sensationalism. Do not become a prey to these superficial swings in food habits, for they are based on economics and your health is never the consideration. A bit of intuitive know how and a lot of commonsense can steer you to a healthy way of eating for a more beautiful you.

One of the most glaring bad food habits that exist today is subsistence on hastily prepared foods or convenience foods as they are called. These are semi-processed add-some-water-type of preparations. Thus, essential minerals are robbed from your food. Today's staple diet consists of foods that are used as snacks. Lack of time, or rather the lack of priority in one's life are the reasons why one so often picks up bad eating habits. If you plan ahead, and educate yourself about the nutritive values of common day-to-day food products, you can eat well and grow beautiful. Let your body "talk" about the food it needs.

There is also a need to dispel some myths about food, nutrients and diet. Some believe that the key to health and beauty is by increasing the daily dose of vitamins. So popping pills becomes a common everyday occurrence. You may not even need to take pills unless you are short on any particular vitamin that you may need to supplement. Mindless pill popping is harmful. Excess is worse than deficiency.

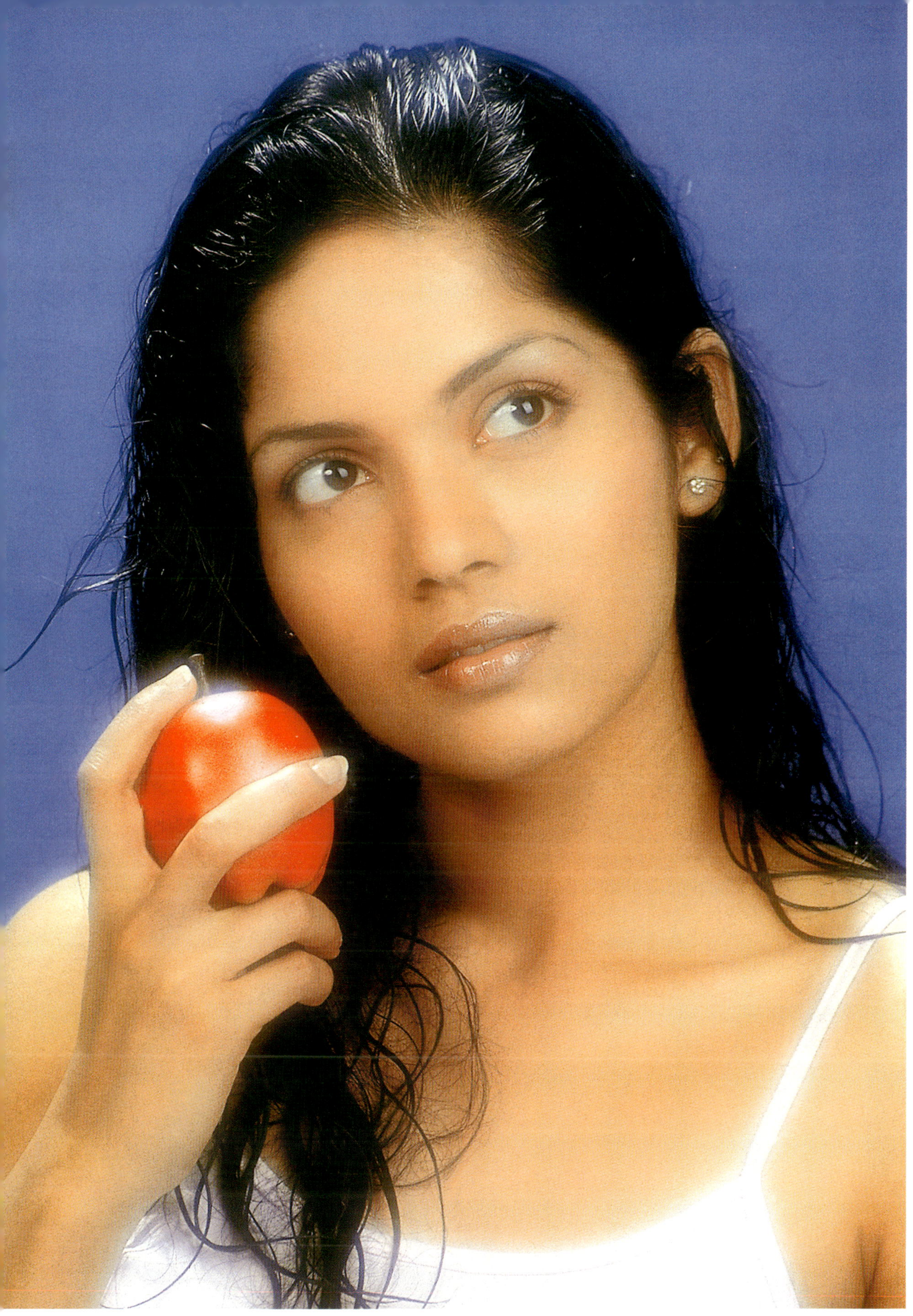

kitchen

A Treasure Trove

Nature has been very generous with its bounty of fruits, flowers, vegetables and herbs. It gives us all that we need to look beautiful, remain healthy and stay youthful.

The early Egyptians were the first to take an interest in using plants for making perfumes and cosmetics. They perhaps learnt the art from the Mesolithic travellers who roamed the Nile valley in 5,000 to 10,000 BC.

The Egyptians had a cure and a preparation for every part of the body. Ancient Egyptian women improved and enhanced their appearances with a variety of cosmetics made from the Earth's bounty.

A judicious use of nature's gifts helps you to enhance your assets and improve upon your drawbacks. It certainly makes you aware that beauty and health are intertwined. Good nutrition and use of natural beauty aids can radiate that aura of beauty that was dormant within you. With the use of these fruits, vegetables, flowers and herbs, you can improve the quality of your hair, texture of your skin and in fact rejuvenate yourself completely.

Health and confidence will reflect not only on your face but also in your complete personality. So, go ahead and make yourself beautiful, not by putting layers of make-up but by enhancing the quality of your skin; hair, and complexion. And by, being content and happy with the way you look naturally. Be beautiful and happy from within.

We owe it to ourselves to spend a little time and effort to grow beautiful. Equipped with these helpful hints from skincare; hair care, face care to nutritional guidelines, you can discover ways to improve your looks and remain youthful and beautiful.

Before you decide on a course of self-improvement, you first need to do a thorough body-check. Recognise your weak beauty points and set about the task of improving upon them and enhancing them. Every product cannot give you a miraculous cure. Using products to improve and enhance yourself has to be a determined and deliberate effort, and it has to fit into a normal routine of your lifestyle. Decide what is best for you; what enhancers you really need and then go about using them regularly to show results and maintain them.

When you are young, you have enough time and spare cash to look after yourself. But as you take on responsibilities of home, hearth and children, beauty care need not take a back seat for want of time or money, if you use the products so easily available in your own kitchen.

Today, beauty houses the world over are being compelled to go back to nature; to use more natural products in their preparations. The modern woman is going back to nature, both in her eating habits and for her body care. Homemade natural beauty aids can prove to be effective if used correctly and consistently.

As you would have realized after going through the beauty care suggestions; fruits, flowers, herbs and vegetables provide cures for improving the quality of the skin, giving a glow to a tired face, imparting health, colour and body to your hair, thus imparting a sense of well-being to the complete body. True, these beauty cures do not have a shelf life, as they contain no preservatives or chemicals. However, you just need to analyse what you need to use everyday, or every week. Once you establish a routine, the task of making and using them is worth the effort of making hem fresh. So, spare a little time for yourself.

Let us now take a look at what your beauty treasure trove in the kitchen has to offer. Indeed your kitchen is like an eco-friendly cosmetic laboratory. It provides you with beauty aids for almost every problem and helps you to overcome flaws, if any, and to enhance your beauty. These cures usually have no side effects and instead beautify you from within and not merely superficially.

Let us now recapitulate some of the most easily available beauty cure aids available right here in your kitchen:

ALMOND : The juice of almonds, crushed and powdered, are extensively used to make face packs, skin nourishers and night creams that nourish and 'feed' your skin. They are extremely useful on aged or wrinkled skins. Usually mixed with rose water and glycerin to make skin nourishers. When added to milk, makes an excellent mask that nourishes and softens your skin.

APPLE : Apple juice if mixed with vinegar makes an excellent hair rinse. Grated apple paste mixed with honey or milk makes an excellent facemask, very useful for complexion cures.

APRICOT : Fresh apricots blended with honey or milk; or fresh apricot paste by itself makes excellent face-masks, which is a very effective nourisher for dry skin, chapped arms, and it helps in rejuvenating dead skin.

AVOCADO : This is a universal favourite. The pulp of this fruit is a skin nourisher and provides an excellent 'food' for the skin. If added to honey or curds, it makes an excellent moisturizer.

BANANA : Pulp if mixed with milk, honey or curds makes a good face-mask that rids you of blemishes. An excellent skin softener. Pulp when mixed with curd and beaten to a thick paste is excellent for your hair, promotes healthy, glossy hair and gives them a unique shine.

CARROT : The ideal 'wrinkle fighter'. Raw carrots grated and added to almond oil and honey and applied as a thick mask, fights wrinkles.

CHICKPEA POWDER : Used as a base for different types of face-masks and as a skin softener and exfoliate. It helps to remove dead skin; hair on the arms and blemishes as well as acne.

COCONUT OIL : Used in numerous beauty care aids. Excellent hair nourisher.

CUCUMBER : Some of the best skin preparations are made from cucumber. When used with curds, makes good, nourishing complexion masks. When used by itself, its juices remove dark circles and blemishes. An excellent skin tautener; it also closes pores, fights skin tan and helps in rejuvenating the skin.

GARLIC: Good for its medicinal properties. If taken raw, it purifies the blood, thus giving a clearer complexion. It also heals cuts and wounds, and clears blemishes if its juice is applied.

GRAPEFRUIT : When the fruit is blended with yogurt it makes a good skin tonic. A skin tautener that also cures blemishes and shadows.

HONEY : A pre-requisite for so many skin nourishers; face-masks and skin tonics. If taken daily with lime and warm water, it purifies blood and clears the skin of blemishes.

HENNA : Its leaves are dried and powdered. Used not only to decorate and beautify the palms, it is universally used as a hair conditioner, colorant and nourisher.

LAVENDER : Its flowers are used to make soaps and hair creams. The oils in these flowers promote hair growth. You can make excellent toilet waters from it to soothe tired nerves. Its essential oils are excellent coolants for headaches and migraines.

LEMON : One of the most commonly used ingredients. A perfect all-rounder used for removing skin tans; as a facemask; as an astringent, as a skin toner and lightener. It tautens the skin and removes wrinkles. Useful to fight dandruff and an excellent tonic if imbibed with honey.

LILAC : Its flowers not only yield a wonderful perfume, they make excellent astringents, bath waters, and soothe sunburnt skin.

MARIGOLD : Its flowers are used to make face creams and skin ointments. It is soothing to the eyes too.

ONION : Onion juice can again be used in various beauty cure treatments. Its juice cures pimples, burn scars and is excellent for dandruff problems. It also helps to restore natural hair colour.

OATS : An excellent base for making face packs, exfoliates and is a remarkable skin tightener.

OLIVE : Used to prepare skin creams to nourish the skin. Revives jaded skin and good for dull, lifeless hair.

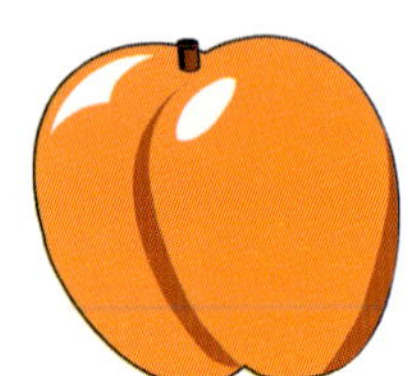

PAPAYA : Again, an excellent and commonly used base for face packs and an excellent hair conditioner. It adds bounce and shine to the hair. The papaya is easily available and its regular use does wonders for your skin and hair.

PEACH : An all time favourite with beauticians all over the world. Makes nourishing facemasks and packs. Fights dry skin and curbs wrinkles. Exfoliates and nourishes.

POTATO : A remarkable skin tautener and helps lighten tan. Heals burns, cuts and lightens your complexion. Helps to get rid of burn marks, removes pimples and freckles.

ROSE : Its petals are used to make a number of beauty preparations and astringents. It softens the skin, fights dry chapped skin and soothes jaded skin.

SAFFRON : Skin enhancer and softener. Excellent for the complexion.

SAGE : Used as a hair colorant. If used with olive oil it also nourishes dry, lifeless hair.

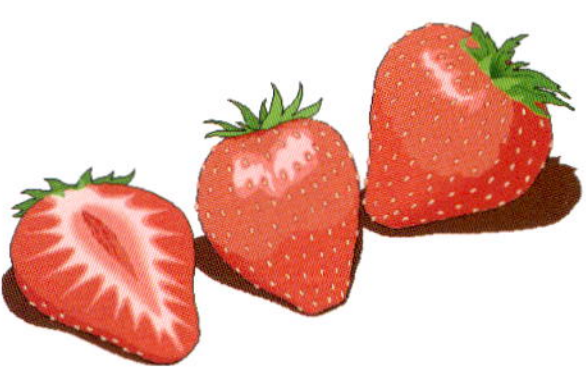

SANDALWOOD : Commonly associated with making perfumes. Its powder when mixed with honey or milk enhances the skin miraculously. It fights tanning; softens the skin and is an excellent cure for pimples, blackheads and blemishes.

STRAWBERRY : Its fruit is crushed and used with milk or honey to make facemasks. Just strawberry juice by itself is an ideal cure for clearing blemishes.

SUNFLOWER : This is also used to cure blemishes.

TURMERIC : Has tremendous curative powers. Cures scars and burn marks. It smoothens the skin and is a base for many other tonics.

TOMATO : Another favourite 'skin toner'. Makes good face masks. A good cleanser and useful for clearing the skin of marks and blemishes.

WALNUT : Both the fruit and its shell are used to darken the hair. Oils extracted from these are used as hair darkeners and mixed with shampoo to give a sheen and gloss and volume to the hair.

WATERCRESS : Used to clear the skin. It smoothens the skin. A paste made from this when applied on burn marks clears them quickly. A good skin hydrator.

WATERMELON : An ideal skin hydrator. It makes the skin taut, refreshed and rehydrated. It also helps to clear shadows under the eyes. There is no better moisturizer than watermelon.

WHEAT : Its husk, or porridge are good exfoliates. Also used as a base in a number of skin mask preparations.

LETTUCE : Makes an excellent astringent. Fights acne and blemishes.

YOGURT : Used in numerous skin preparations to make skincare masks, packs, and by itself as a skin smoothener. Fights acne. Yogurt is also used in a number of hair care preparations. It nourishes the hair, helping in healthy hair growth.

The magical beauty treasure chest in your own kitchen can help you create your own beauty kit. You can remain beautiful and healthy by using these natural beauty aids. Ultimately, we do fall back on nature to help us become truly beautiful. So give yourself a natural makeover from your own kitchen beauty box, which is indeed a treasure trove of beauty aids.

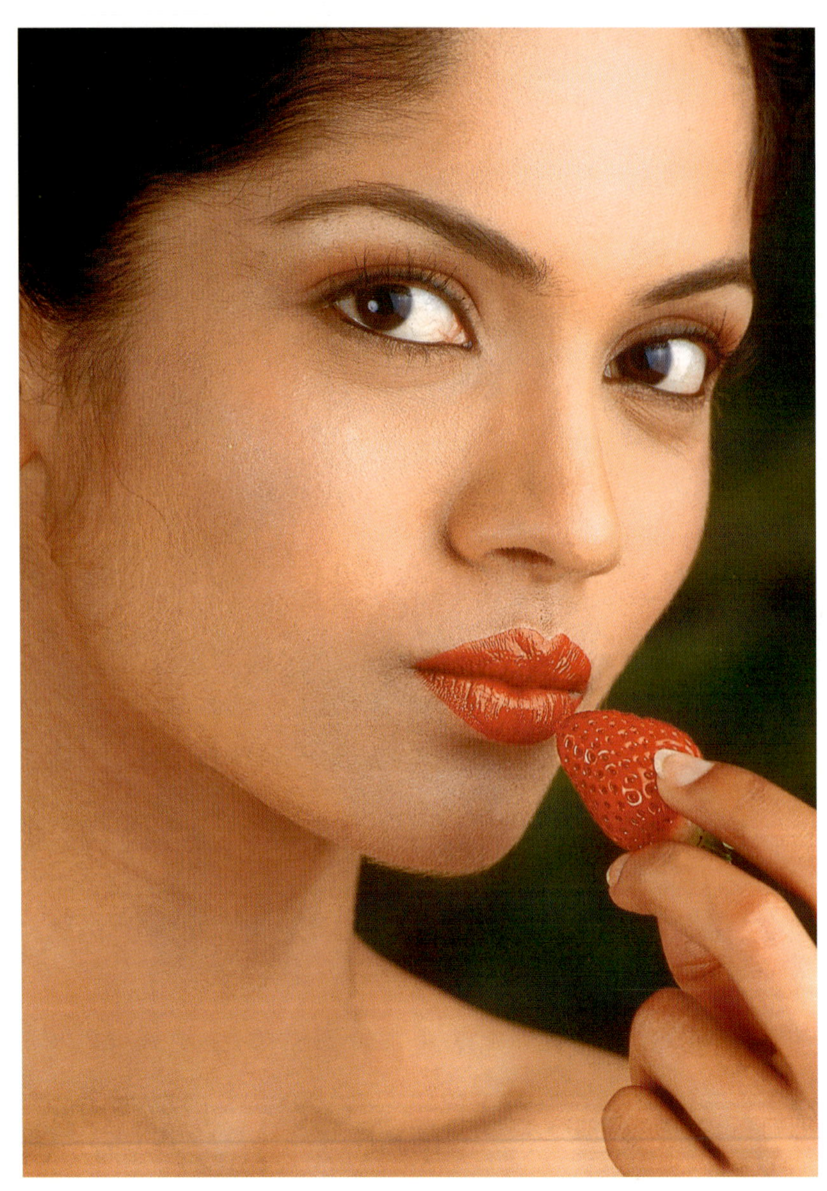